Paleo
for Beginners

Delicious Paleo Diet Recipes

Jamie Evans

TABLE OF CONTENTS

---- BREAKFAST ----

---- LUNCH ----

---- DINNER ----

---- DESSERTS ----

---- SNACKS ----

Breakfast

TURKEY SAUSAGE PATTIES WITH LEMON SPINACH

A quick and healthy breakfast that is filling and nutritious. You can make these patties ahead of time so breakfast comes together in minutes.

MAKES 1 SERVING/ TOTAL TIME 20 MINUTE

INGREDIENTS

1 pound ground turkey

1 egg

1 onion finely diced

2 cloves garlic minced

1 teaspoon paprika

1 teaspoon oregano

1 teaspoon ground sage

2 tablespoons olive oil

1 pound baby spinach

Juice of 1 lemon

Sea salt and fresh ground

pepper to taste

METHOD

STEP 1

Combine the turkey, egg, onion, garlic, and seasonings in a mixing bowl and mix until combined. Form into 2-inch breakfast patties. Heat the oil in a skillet over medium high heat and cook the sausage patties until browned and cooked through. Remove from pan.

STEP 2

Add the spinach and cook until wilted. Add the lemon juice. Serve the sausage with the spinach.

NUTRITION VALUE

354 Kcal, 17g fat, 10g fiber, 33g protein, 14g carbs.

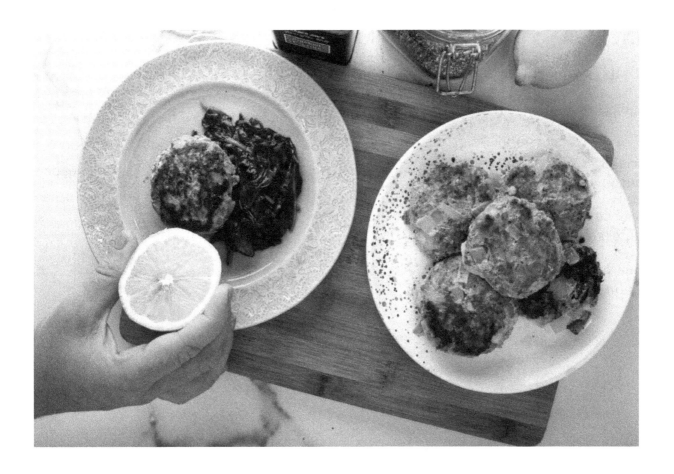

HERBED CHICKEN OMELET

An easy omelet that is loaded with protein and flavored with fresh herbs. Use whatever herbs you like here to customize the flavor.

MAKES 1 SERVING/ TOTAL TIME 10 MINUTE

INGREDIENTS

1 tablespoon butter or olive oil

3 eggs beaten

1/4 cup fresh chopped herbs such as parsley, basil, chives, or rosemary or combination

1/2 cup cooked and shredded chicken breast

Sea salt and fresh ground pepper to taste

METHOD

STEP 1

Heat the butter in a small skillet over medium low heat. Add the eggs and cook for a minute until the edges are set. Lift the edges carefully and let the liquid flow underneath the edges. Season with salt and pepper. Sprinkle the herbs over the omelet, add the chicken and carefully fold in half. Continue cooking until done and serve

NUTRITION VALUE

614 Kcal, 20g fat, 3g fiber, 76g protein, 5g carbs.

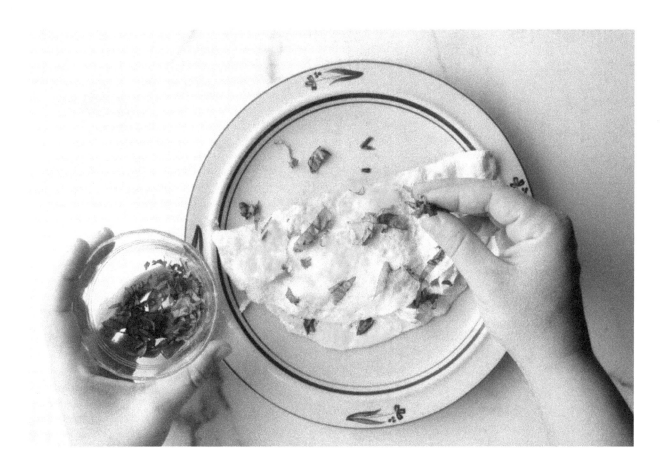

STEAK, EGGS, AND GREENS

A classic breakfast dish gets a nutrient upgrade with the addition of hearty chopped greens. It's the perfect combination of protein, carbs, and fat.

MAKES 2 SERVING/ TOTAL TIME 20 MINUTE

INGREDIENTS

1 tablespoon olive oil

10 ounces beef tenderloin cubed

1 clove garlic minced

1 bunch hearty greens such as kale or collards chopped

1/2 teaspoon crushed red pepper flakes

2 eggs

Sea salt and fresh ground pepper to taste

METHOD

STEP 1
Heat the oil in a heavy nonstick skillet. Add the beef and cook until done to your liking. Remove from pan and add the garlic and greens.

STEP 2
Cook until wilted and add the pepper flakes. Make two wells in the greens and crack the eggs in the pan. Cook to your liking.

Serve with the steak.

NUTRITION VALUE	438 Kcal, 20g fat, 2g fiber, 49g protein, 6g carbs.

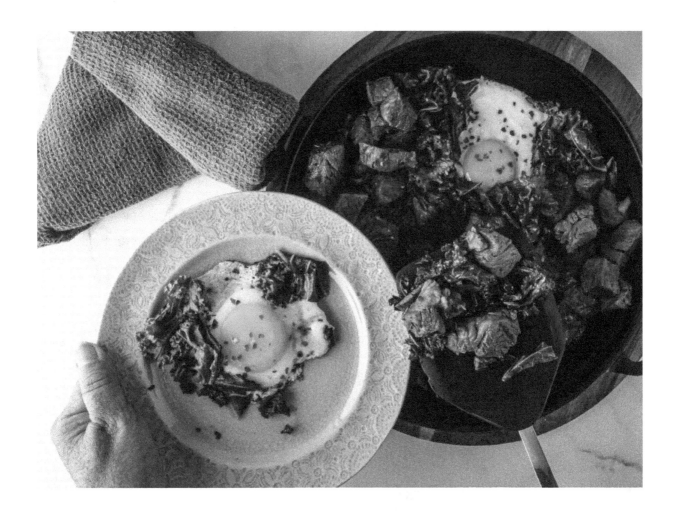

SPINACH AND AVOCADO SCRAMBLE

A quick and easy breakfast that is full of greens and protein, with the addition of the good fat in avocado to keep you full. Perfect when you know you've got a busy day ahead.

MAKES 2 SERVING/ TOTAL TIME 10 MINUTE

INGREDIENTS

1 tablespoon butter or olive oil

1 shallot minced

2 cloves garlic minced

4 cups chopped spinach

6 eggs beaten well

1 avocado diced

Sea salt and fresh ground pepper to taste

METHOD

STEP 1

Heat a large nonstick skillet over medium heat. Add the shallot and garlic and cook until soft. Add the spinach; cook until wilted. Season with salt and pepper.

STEP 2

Add the eggs, and scramble as they cook. When done, divide between two plates and top with the avocado before serving.

NUTRITION VALUE

441 Kcal, 20g fat,
8g fiber, 23g protein, 14.5g carbs.

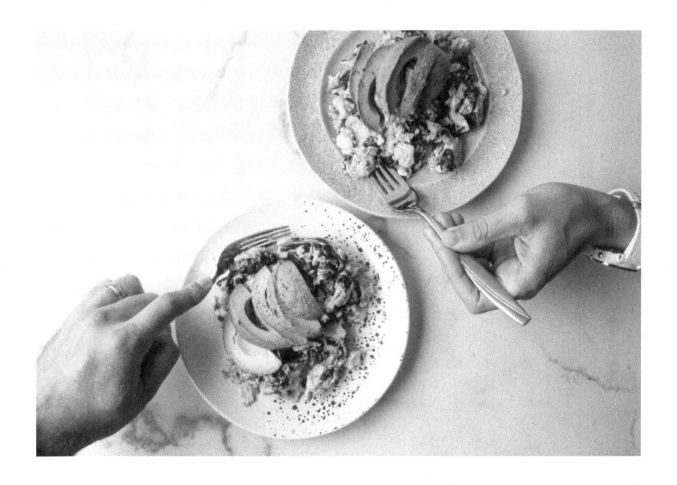

FRIED EGGS WITH CURRIED CAULIFLOWER RICE

A spicy cauliflower rice turns breakfast into an exotic meal. Perfect when you're tired of the same things every day.

MAKES 2 SERVING/ TOTAL TIME 20 MINUTE

INGREDIENTS

1 tablespoon coconut oil

4 cups riced cauliflower

2 teaspoons curry powder

2 tablespoons chopped cilantro

Juice of 1 lime

4 eggs

Sea salt and fresh ground pepper to taste

METHOD

STEP 1

Heat the oil in a large, deep skillet. Add the cauliflower and curry powder and stir until softened. Add the cilantro and lime juice and remove from pan.

STEP 2

Add the eggs to the pan and cook to your liking. Season with salt and pepper and serve with the cauliflower.

NUTRITION VALUE

480Kcal, 17g fat, 19g fiber, 20g protein, 14.6g carbs.

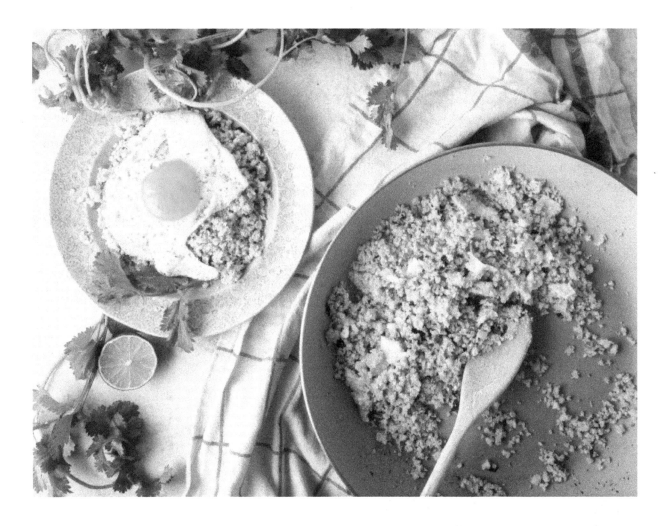

BACON AND ASPARAGUS OMELET

Tender asparagus pairs beautifully with bacon, and when wrapped up in a fluffy omelet, it makes breakfast that is healthy, nutritious and delicious.

MAKES 1 SERVING/ TOTAL TIME 10 MINUTE

INGREDIENTS

2 slices bacon diced

5 stalks asparagus chopped

3 eggs beaten

2 tablespoons grated Parmesan cheese

Sea salt and fresh ground pepper to taste

METHOD

STEP 1

Cook the bacon in a nonstick skillet and remove with a slotted spoon. Add the asparagus to the pan and cook until tender. Remove and add to the bacon, leaving as much fat behind as you can.

STEP 2

Add the eggs and cook for a minute until the edges are set. Lift the edges carefully and let the liquid flow underneath the edges. Top with the bacon, asparagus and Parmesan. Carefully fold in half and continue cooking until eggs are done.

Slide onto a plate and serve.

NUTRITION VALUE	348 Kcal, 20g fat, 2g fiber, 28g protein, 5g carbs.

Lunch

PORK CUTLETS WITH BABY TRUSS TOMATOES

Take one baking tray, add ingredients, slide it into a warm oven and let the flavors mingle as meat becomes golden and vegies turn crisp on the outside and tender on the inside.

MAKES 6 SERVING/ TOTAL TIME 50 MINUTE

INGREDIENTS

6 pork cutlets

2 tablespoons Cajun seasoning

1 tablespoon olive oil

1 large red onion, halved, cut into wedges

6 Lebanese eggplants, halved lengthways

3 **zucchini**, quartered lengthways

Olive oil spray

2 red apples, halved, cored, cut into thick wedges

2 x 275g pkts baby roma truss tomatoes

METHOD

STEP 1

Preheat oven to 200°C. Sprinkle both sides of pork with the seasoning. Heat the oil in a large heavy-based flameproof roasting pan over medium heat. Cook the pork for 2 minutes each side or until golden. Transfer to a plate.

STEP 2

Place the onion, eggplant and zucchini in the pan. Spray with oil and season with salt and pepper. Roast for 15 minutes or until the vegetables just start to soften.

STEP 3

Arrange the pork, apple and tomatoes in the pan with the vegetables. Roast, using a spoon to remove any excess liquid from the pan halfway through cooking, for a further 20 minutes.

NUTRITION VALUE

1028 KJ Energy, 9g fat, 1g saturated fat, 5g fiber, 33g protein, 12g carbs.

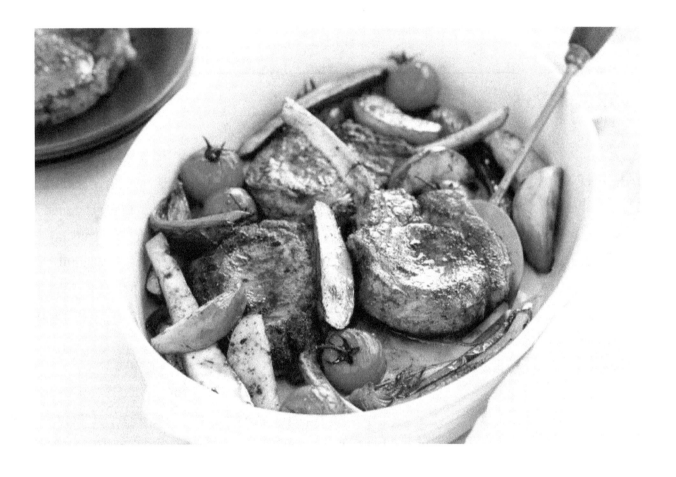

PALEO ALMOND, PECAN AND COCONUT CRUMBED CHICKEN

Baked chicken with a nutty, crunchy coating served with a warm vege salad ticks all the boxes for a healthy, Paleo-friendly meal.

MAKES 4 SERVING/ TOTAL TIME 50 MINUTE

INGREDIENTS

1/2 cup natural almonds

1/3 cup pecans

1/2 cup shredded coconut

3 teaspoons lemon rind,

1 garlic clove, quartered

1 egg, lightly beaten

1 tablespoon water, cold

4 small **Chicken Breasts**

1 tablespoon macadamia oil

250g Brussels sprouts,

1 large head broccoli,

1 tablespoon pine nuts

1 tablespoon pepitas

1 tablespoon sunflower kernels

1/2 avocado, roughly chopped

1/4 cup apple cider vinegar

2 tablespoons macadamia oil

1 teaspoon Dijon mustard

METHOD
STEP 1
Preheat oven to 180C/160C fan-forced. Line a baking tray with baking paper. Process almonds, pecans, coconut, lemon rind and garlic in a food processor until finely chopped. Transfer to a large shallow bowl. Season with salt and pepper. Whisk egg and water in a shallow bowl until combined. Dip chicken in egg mixture, then press in nut mixture to coat all over. Transfer to prepared tray. Drizzle with oil. Bake for 30 minutes
STEP 2
Meanwhile, make Broccoli and sprout salad: Cook Brussels sprouts in a large saucepan of boiling water for 2 minutes or until just starting to turn bright green. Transfer to a large bowl of iced water. Repeat with broccoli. Heat a small frying pan over medium high heat. Cook pine nuts, pepitas and sunflower seeds for 3 to 4 minutes or until toasted. Drain sprouts and broccoli. Transfer to a large bowl. Add avocado and pine nut mixture. Whisk vinegar, oil, mustard and dill in a jug. Season with salt and pepper. Drizzle over salad.

NUTRITION VALUE

1190 KJ Energy, 20g fat, 7g fiber, 46.8g protein, 5.8g carbs.

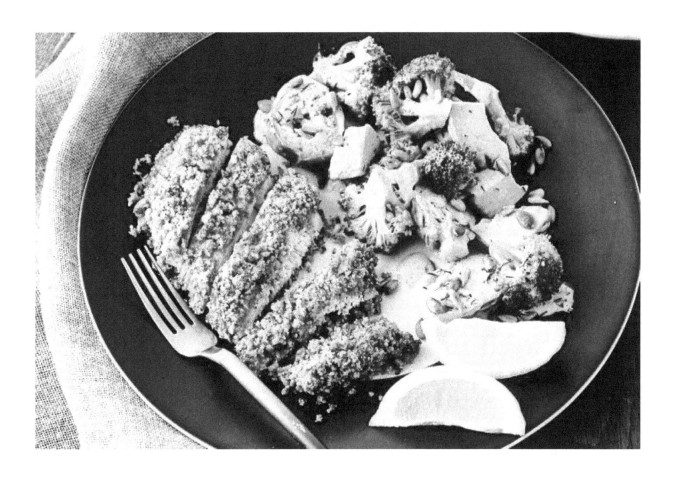

PORK AND SWEET POTATO SKEWERS

Recipe that everyone love.

MAKES 4 SERVING/ TOTAL TIME 65 MINUTE

INGREDIENTS

500g orange sweet potato, peeled, cubed

600g **pork fillet**, cubed

2 tbsp olive oil

1 tbsp ground cumin

1/3 cup wholegrain mustard

Chopped chives, to serve

Apple sauce, to serve

METHOD

STEP 1

Place potato and 2 tablespoons water in a heatproof, microwave-safe bowl. Microwave, covered, on high (100%) for 4 to 5 minutes or until just tender. Drain. Set aside to cool.

STEP 2

Thread pork and potato onto 8 skewers. Place in a dish. Drizzle with oil. Sprinkle with cumin. Turn to coat.

STEP 3

Preheat a barbecue plate or chargrill on medium heat. Cook skewers, turning occasionally, for 6 to 8 minutes or until pork is cooked through and potato is browned. Remove to a plate. Set aside, covered, for 5 minutes to rest.

STEP 4

Brush skewers with mustard. Sprinkle with chives. Serve with apple sauce.

NUTRITION VALUE

1450 KJ Energy, 12g fat, 2g saturated fat, 3 fiber, 37 Protein, 12g carbs.

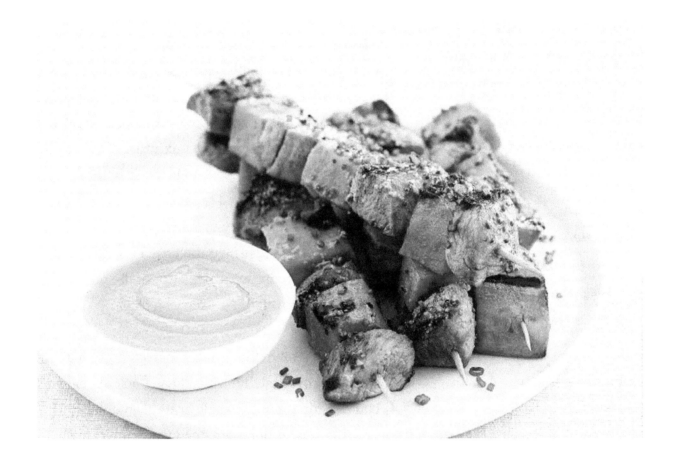

PORK AND EGGPLANT PARMIGIANA

This tasty pork and eggplant parmigiana recipe can be made ahead of time and will have all the family asking for more!

MAKES 1 SERVING/ TOTAL TIME 10 MINUTE

INGREDIENTS

1 cup (75g) panko breadcrumbs

1/4 cup (20g) finely grated parmesan

1 garlic clove, crushed

1 tbs flat-leaf parsley, finely chopped

2 Coles Australian Free-Range Eggs, lightly whisked

2 x 400g pkts Coles Australian Pork Sizzle Steak*

Olive oil, to shallow-fry

1 large eggplant, sliced crossways

500g Coles Mum's Sause Garden Veg

200g mozzarella, sliced

Green salad, to serve

METHOD

STEP 1

Place the breadcrumbs, parmesan, garlic and parsley in a shallow bowl and stir to combine. Season. Place the egg in a separate shallow bowl. Dip 1 pork steak in the egg, then in the breadcrumb mixture and turn to coat. Transfer to a plate. Repeat, in batches, with the remaining pork, egg and breadcrumb mixture. Add enough oil to a large frying pan to come 1cm up the side of the pan. Heat over medium heat. Cook the pork, in batches, for 3 mins each side or until the pork is golden and cooked through. Transfer to a plate.

STEP 2

Add enough oil to the frying pan to come 1cm up the side. Heat over medium-high heat. Cook the eggplant, in batches, for 1 min each side or until golden brown. Transfer to another plate lined with paper towel. Preheat grill on high. Line a large baking tray with foil. Place the pork on the lined tray. Spoon the pasta sauce evenly over the pork. Top with the eggplant and mozzarella. Cook under the grill for 5 mins or until mozzarella melts and is golden. Divide the pork mixture and salad evenly among serving plates. Season.

NUTRITION VALUE

1937 KJ Energy, 20g fat, 7g saturated fat, 3g fiber, 45g protein, 15g carbs.

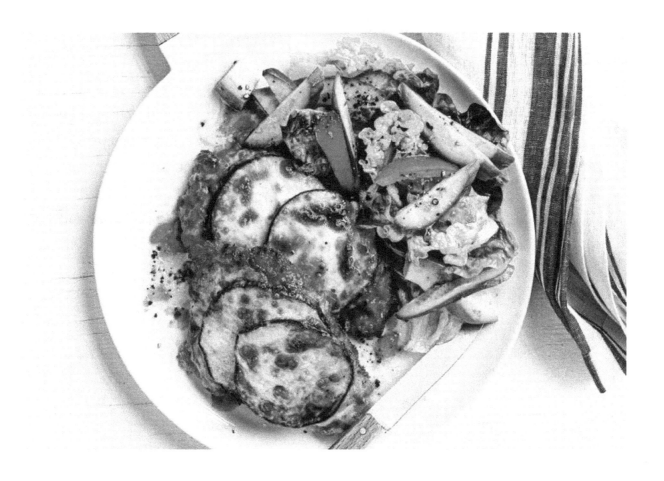

SALMON WITH MANGO & CHILLI SALSA

Bursting with goodness, this low-fat recipe fuses sweet fruit with fresh vegies - perfect for a warm **summer** day or evening.

MAKES 4 SERVING/ TOTAL TIME 25 MINUTE

INGREDIENTS

1 tbsp olive oil

4 (about 220g each) skinless **salmon** fillets

2 ripe mangoes, cheeks removed, peeled, finely chopped

1 long fresh red chili, halved, deseeded, thinly sliced

2 tbsp chopped fresh coriander

1 tbsp fresh lime juice

1 bunch asparagus, woody ends trimmed

Lime wedges, to serve

METHOD

STEP 1

Heat oil in a non-stick frying pan over medium-high heat. Season salmon with salt and pepper. Cook for 3-4 minutes each side or until just cooked through.

STEP 2

Meanwhile, combine the mango, chili, coriander and lime juice in a bowl. Taste and season with salt and pepper.

STEP 3

Cook the asparagus in a saucepan of boiling water for 2-3 minutes or until bright green and tender crisp.

STEP 4

Divide the salmon among serving plates. Top with asparagus and salsa and serve with lime wedges.

NUTRITION VALUE

2100 KJ Energy, 20g fat, 5g saturated fat, 2g fiber, 55g protein, 11g carbs.

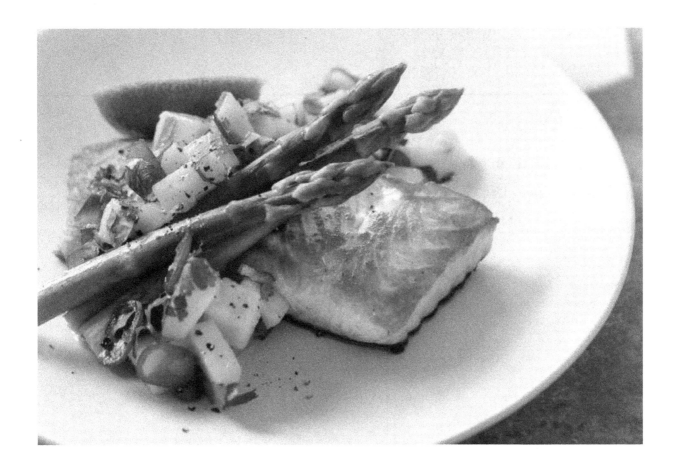

ROAST CHICKEN THIGH FILLETS

Use these tasty roast chicken thighs as a base for some great family meals such as stir-fries, pastas and pies.

MAKES 8 SERVING/ TOTAL TIME 25 MINUTE

INGREDIENTS

8 x 150g **chicken thigh** fillets

2 tablespoons olive oil

METHOD

STEP 1

Preheat oven to 180°C/160°C fan-forced. Place chicken in a large roasting pan. Drizzle with oil. Toss to coat chicken in oil. Season with salt and pepper.

STEP 2

Roast for 20 minutes or until chicken is cooked through. Allow to cool before refrigerating.

NUTRITION VALUE

1081 KJ Energy, 17g fat, 4g saturated fat, 26g protein, 13.5g carbs.

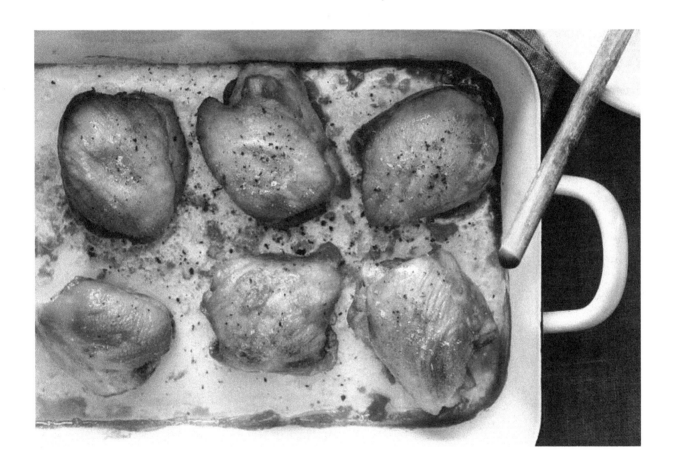

OLIVE & HERB FISH PARCELS

Recipe that Everyone love.

MAKES 4 SERVING/ TOTAL TIME 20 MINUTE

INGREDIENTS

120g baby spinach leaves

4 blue-eye fillets, deboned

2 **zucchini**, sliced

40 small black olives

120ml extra virgin olive oil

2 tablespoons lemon juice

2 teaspoons grated lemon rind

1 garlic clove, finely chopped

1 tablespoon finely chopped mint

2 tablespoons finely chopped basil

1 tablespoon finely chopped chives

METHOD

STEP 1

Preheat the oven to 190°C.

STEP 2

Cut four 30cm sheets of foil and lay on work surface. Cut 4 sheets of baking paper the same size and place on top of foil.

STEP 3

Divide spinach between parcels, then place a fish fillet on top. Divide zucchini and olives between parcels. Use a total of 2 tablespoons of the olive oil to drizzle onto fish. Season with salt and pepper.

STEP 4

Place remaining oil in a small bowl, whisk in lemon juice and rind, garlic and fresh herbs, then season with salt and pepper. Pour a little of the mixture over each fillet, bring up the edges and seal.

STEP 5

Bake for 10 minutes or until fish is cooked through - it will flake away easily when tested with a fork. Drizzle with remaining dressing, and serve with boiled chat potatoes, if desired.

NUTRITION VALUE

1735 KJ Energy, 20g fat, 3g saturated fat, 3g fiber, 21g protein, 3g carbs.

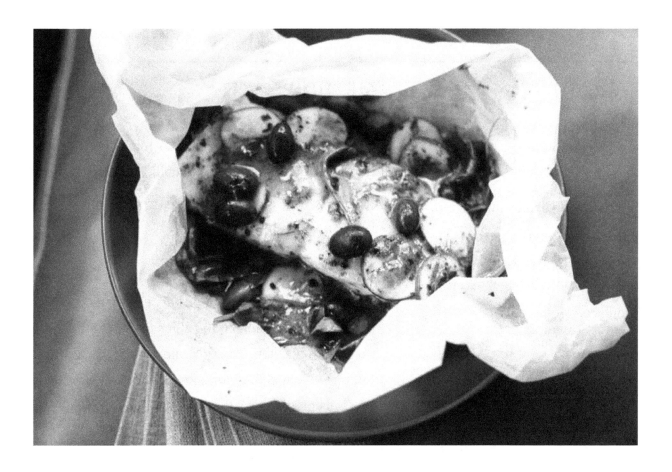

KINGFISH SKEWERS WITH CHARGRILLED TOMATOES AND CHILLIES

These gluten-free kingfish skewers make a light and lovely lunch.

MAKES 4 SERVING/ TOTAL TIME 35 MINUTE

INGREDIENTS

1/4 cup (60ml) lemon juice

5-6 parsley sprigs, leaves roughly chopped

1/2 teaspoon dried chili flakes

1 1/2 tablespoons olive oil

800g skinless kingfish fillets, pin boned, cut into 3cm cubes

3 long red chilies

3 long green chilies

250g vine-ripened cherry tomatoes

METHOD

STEP 1

Soak 8 wooden skewers in water for 10 minutes. Combine juice, parsley, dried chili, 2 teaspoons oil and fish in a bowl. Cover and refrigerate for 10 minutes, then thread onto skewers.

STEP 2

Meanwhile, toss chilies and tomatoes in remaining olive oil. Heat an oiled chargrill or barbecue over medium-high heat. When hot, cook chilies for 10 minutes, turning to blacken. The skin should pop and crack open. Cut open each chili down one side and remove seeds (unless you like it really spicy).

STEP 3

Add the kingfish skewers to the chargrill or barbecue and cook for 6-8 minutes, turning once, or until just cooked. Add the tomatoes and cook for the final 5 minutes, or until softened and lightly charred. Serve 2 skewers per person with chargrilled tomatoes and chilies.

NUTRITION VALUE

1240 KJ Energy, 11.7g fat, 2.6g saturated fat, 2.4g fiber, 42.6g protein, 3.1g carbs.

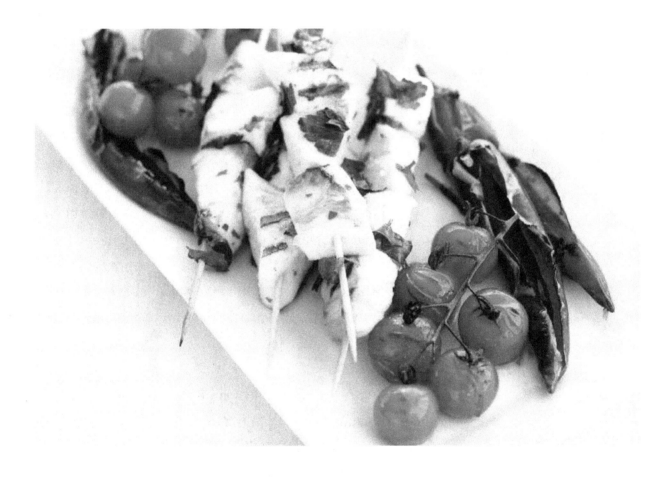

CHICKEN WITH LEMON AND GARLIC

Lemon and garlic add flavor to the **chicken** as well as ensuring it is extra juicy.

MAKES 4 SERVING/ TOTAL TIME 35 MINUTE

INGREDIENTS

4 **chicken Maryland** pieces

2 teaspoons thyme leaves

1 tablespoon finely grated lemon rind

2 cloves garlic, crushed

85g unsalted butter, softened

METHOD

STEP 1

Pre-heat oven to 220°C. Place the lemon rind, butter, garlic, thyme leaves, salt and pepper in a bowl and mix until combined. Set aside.

STEP 2

Using your fingers or the back of a teaspoon, push deeply but gently between the skin and flesh of each chicken Maryland piece to separate them and form a pocket. Divide the lemon butter mixture between four chicken thighs, pushing the butter evenly down towards the drumstick. Wipe any remaining butter over the surface of the chicken skin.

STEP 3

Place the chicken in a large baking dish lined with baking paper. Scatter a few extra thyme sprigs in the dish. Bake for 25 minutes, basting regularly until golden. Serve with steamed vegetables.

NUTRITION VALUE

1617 KJ Energy, 20g fat, 1g fiber, 35g protein, 14.9g carbs.

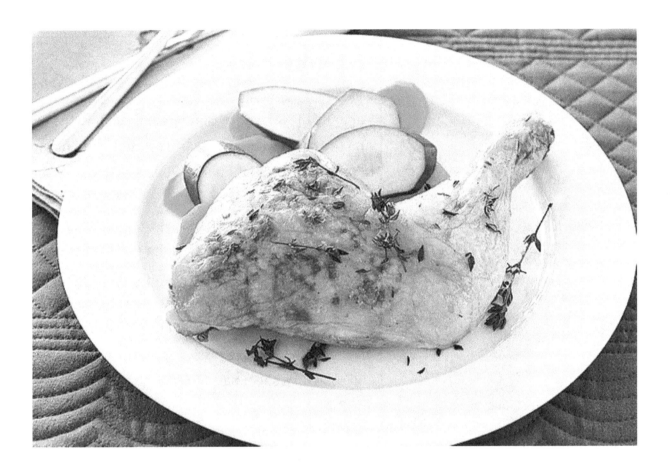

INSTANT POT BRISKET TACO BOWLS

Briny brisket all seasoned up, then shredded to crispy perfection. Nuzzled up to some spiced cauliflower rice, shredded lettuce and avocado.

MAKES 3 SERVING/ TOTAL TIME 1 HOUR 17 MINUTE

INGREDIENTS

2-pound brisket

2 teaspoons fine salt

2 tablespoons mustard seeds

2 bay leaves

1 teaspoon nutmeg

1 tablespoon cumin

1 tablespoon garlic powder

2 tablespoons grated beetroot

3 tablespoons vinegar

3 cups bone broth plus water

16 ounces cauliflower rice

2 tablespoons avocado oil

1 teaspoon turmeric

1 teaspoon garlic salt

1 teaspoon dried oregano

METHOD

STEP 1

Combine the brisket seasonings and rub into the meat. Add the beetroot and vinegar. Toss and set to marinate in the fridge for 30 minutes. When ready to cook, heat the pressure cooker on sauté mode. When hot, add the brisket, fatty side down and sear for 2 minutes, then flip and sear the other side. Cancel the sauce function. Add in the bone broth, then enough water to submerge the brisket. Pour in any leftover marinade. Set to pressure cook on high for 50 minutes. Release the pressure manually. Remove the brisket from the pressure cooker and set it on a sheet pan. Shred with two forks.

STEP 2

Place the oven rack right under the broiler. Heat the broiler at 500F.

Spread the brisket out over half of the sheet pan and spoon a little liquid from the pressure cooker over it. On the other half of the sheet pan toss the cauliflower rice with avocado oil and seasoning and spread out flat on the sheet pan. To make your bowls, distribute the cauliflower rice and brisket. Add shredded lettuce, avocado, cilantro and green onion.

NUTRITION VALUE	806 Kcal, 20g fat, 10g fiber, 79g protein, 14g carbs.

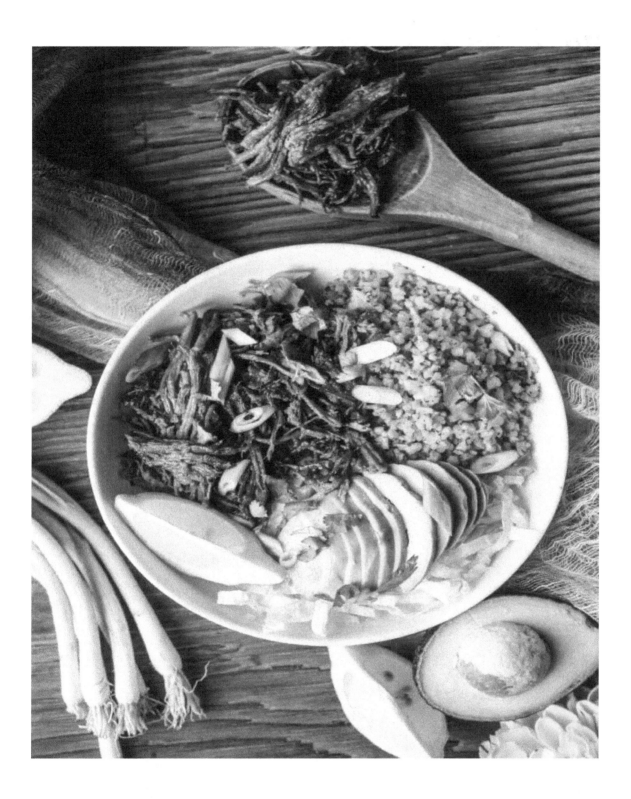

PALEO JAMBALAYA

The following recipe will set you out on a hunt for the best andouille sausages you can find.

MAKES 4 SERVING/ TOTAL TIME 35 MINUTE

INGREDIENTS

2 tbsp. olive oil

1 lb. Andouille sausages, sliced

2 lbs. chicken tenders,

1 onion, chopped3 cloves garlic, minced

3 celery stalks, chopped

1 green bell pepper, sliced

1 red bell pepper, sliced

4 fresh thyme sprigs

2 cups chicken broth

1 cup tomato sauce

1/4 cup hot sauce (optional)

1 lb. raw shrimp,

8 oz. okra, chopped

2 tbsp. parsley, finely chopped

4 green onions, chopped

METHOD

STEP 1

In a large saucepan over high heat, brown the sausages in the olive oil. Cook for approximately 3 minutes, or until golden brown.

Add the chicken to the saucepan and season with salt and pepper. Continue cooking on all sides for a few more minutes until the chicken begins to brown.

STEP 2

Add the onion, garlic, celery, peppers and thyme to the saucepan. Mix in with the meat and continue to cook for 5 to 7 minutes; stirring frequently to prevent anything from sticking to the bottom of the pan.

Add the broth, tomato sauce and hot sauce. Mix well and allow it to come to a boil.

Once the mixture has boiled, add the shrimp and okra. Reduce the heat and simmer, covered, for 5 to 7 minutes, or until shrimp is pink.

Remove the jambalaya from the heat. Stir in parsley and green onions prior to serving.

NUTRITION VALUE

800 Kcal, 20g fat, 57g protein, 13g carbs.

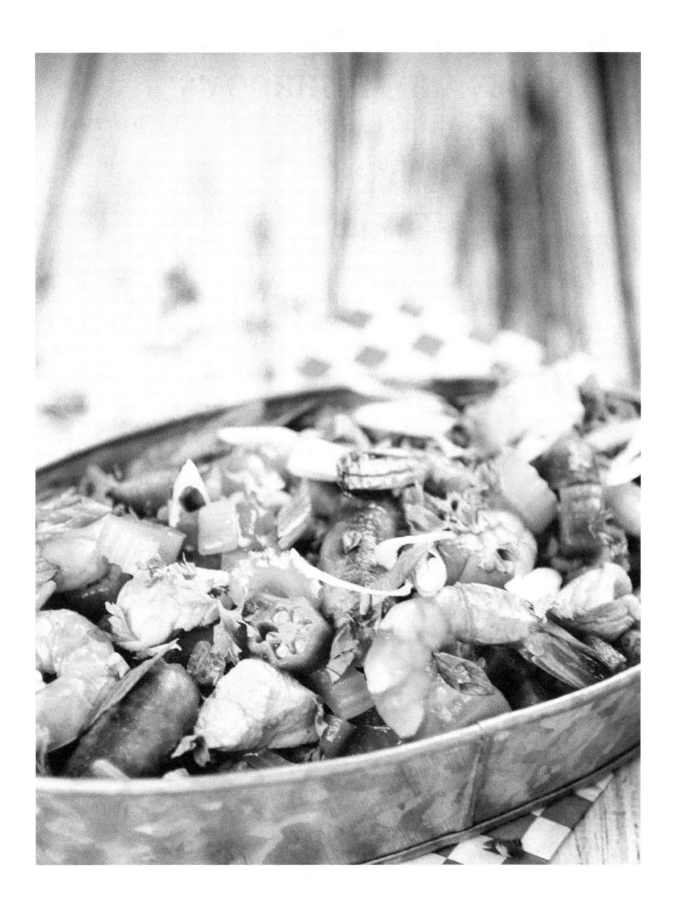

CHICKEN WITH SPINACH, SWEET POTATOES AND MUSHROOMS

Chicken often makes a delightful appearance with mashed **sweet potatoes** and green vegetables.

MAKES 4 SERVING/ TOTAL TIME 60 MINUTE

INGREDIENTS

2 lbs. chicken breasts, skinless, boneless and sliced

2 sweet potatoes, peeled and diced

10 mushrooms, sliced

1 red onion, sliced

2 garlic cloves, minced

2 cups baby spinach

1/2 cup chicken stock

1 cup coconut milk

1 tbsp. garlic powder

1 tbsp. onion powder

1 tbsp. paprika

1 tbsp. coconut oil

METHOD

STEP 1

Preheat oven to 375 F. In a bowl, combine the garlic powder, onion powder and paprika, then season to taste. Season the chicken pieces with the spice mixture. Melt the coconut oil in a skillet over medium-high heat. Brown the chicken in the skillet on both sides, 2 to 3 minutes per side; then transfer to a baking dish.

Cook the diced sweet potatoes for 5 to 6 minutes in the skillet over medium heat. Add more coconut oil if needed.

STEP 2

Add the onion, mushrooms, and garlic to the sweet potatoes and cook for another 2 to 3 minutes.

Add the sweet potatoes, onion, mushrooms, and garlic to the baking dish.

Pour in the coconut milk and chicken stock.

Top with baby spinach, give everything a toss.

Place in the oven and bake for 18 to 20 minutes, covered. Bake another 10 minutes uncovered.

NUTRITION VALUE 20g fat, 74g protein, 15g carbs.

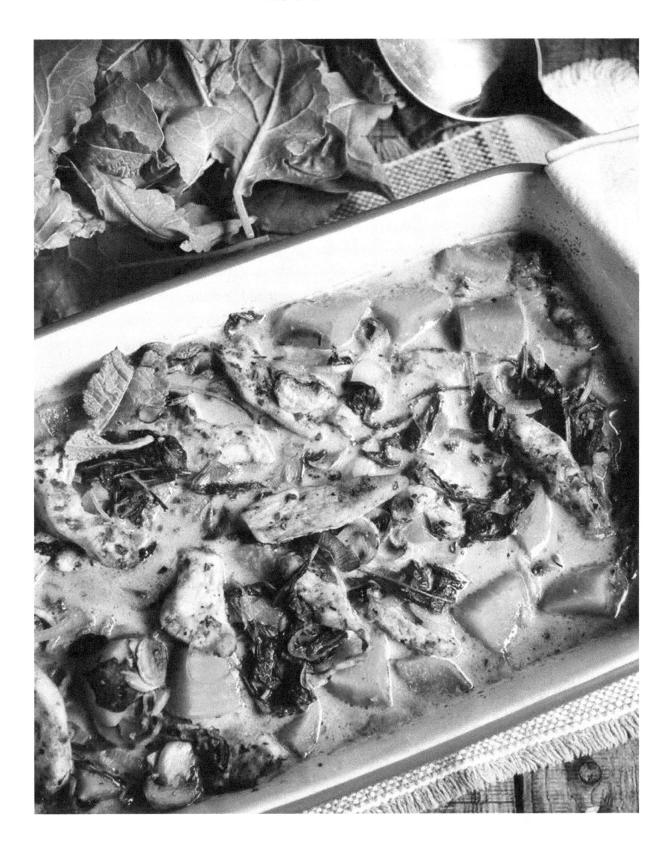

CURRIED MANGO SHRIMP KEBOBS

Sweet and spicy, these easy kebobs will be the hit of your next backyard barbecue. Make them up in advance and then grill when ready to eat.

MAKES 4 SERVING/ TOTAL TIME 20 MINUTE

INGREDIENTS

1-pound raw shrimp

2 cups diced mango

1 tablespoon melted coconut oil

1 teaspoon curry powder

METHOD

STEP 1

Thread the shrimp and mango onto skewers. Brush with coconut oil and sprinkle with curry powder.

STEP 2

Preheat a gas or charcoal grill to medium high heat. Grill until shrimp is pink and mango is lightly charred. Serve

NUTRITION VALUE

162 Kcal, 5g fat,
2g fiber, 20g protein, 14g carbs.

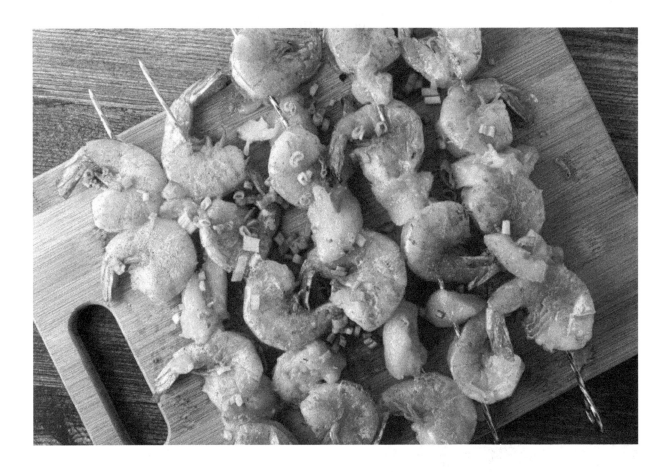

BACON MUSHROOM THYME BURGERS

Loaded with salty bacon and mushrooms, these burgers are so delicious, you won't miss the bun!

MAKES 4 SERVING/ TOTAL TIME 20 MINUTE

INGREDIENTS

1 pound ground beef

1 egg

1 cup finely chopped mushrooms

1 teaspoon fresh thyme leaves

4 slices bacon cooked and crumbled

Sea salt and fresh ground pepper to taste

METHOD

STEP 1

Combine the beef, egg, mushroom, thyme and bacon with a pinch of salt and pepper. Form into 4 patties.

STEP 2

Preheat a gas or charcoal grill to medium heat. Grill the burgers until done to your liking and serve with your favorite toppings.

NUTRITION VALUE

266Kcal, 17g fat, 28g protein, 1g carbs.

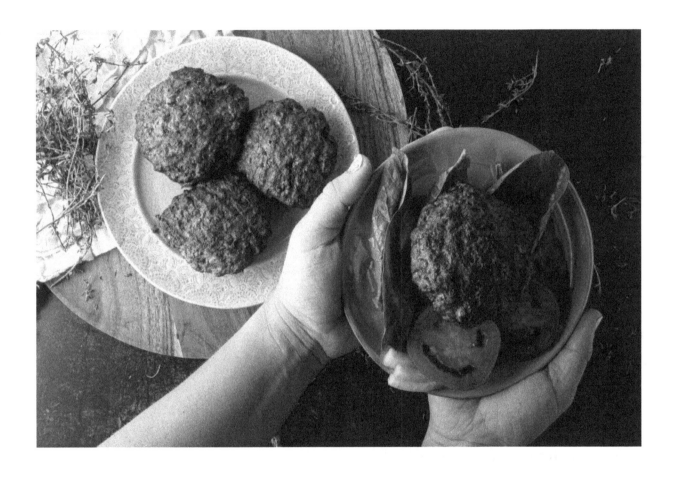

DIJON HERB CHICKEN SALAD

Lots of herbs and a garlic mustard dressing turn traditional chicken salad into a new, exciting dish. It's creamy, flavorful, and delicious, while still being nutritious and filling — a win when it comes to lunch!

MAKES 2 SERVING/ TOTAL TIME 15 MINUTE

INGREDIENTS

1/4 cup plain Greek yogurt

1 tablespoon Dijon mustard

2 cloves garlic minced

1 teaspoon apple cider vinegar

2 tablespoons chopped fresh parsley

1 tablespoon chopped thyme leaves

1 tablespoon chopped rosemary leaves

2 cups cooked and shredded chicken breast

1 red onion sliced

Lettuce leaves or spinach for serving

Sea salt and fresh ground pepper to taste

METHOD

STEP 1

Whisk the yogurt, mustard, garlic, and cider vinegar in a bowl. Add the remaining ingredients and mix well.

Chill until ready to serve.

Serve in the lettuce leaves or over a bed of spinach.

NUTRITION VALUE

459 Kcal, 10g fat, 3g fiber, 73g protein, 14.9g carbs.

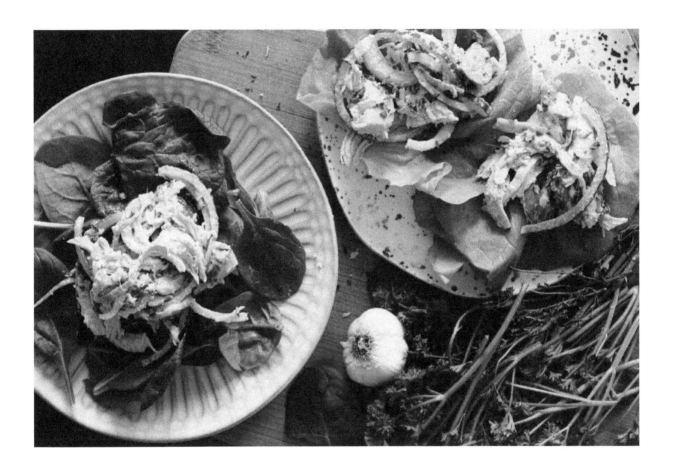

Dinner

CAJUN CHICKEN WITH AVOCADO, LIME AND CHILLI SALSA

Spice up your weeknight night with this healthy, low-carb Cajun chicken dish.

MAKES 4 SERVING/ TOTAL TIME 28 MINUTE

INGREDIENTS

4 small (180g each) **chicken breast** fillets

1 tbsp sweet paprika

Pinch of cayenne pepper

1 avocado, flesh cubed

2 tbsp lime juice

1 long green chili, seeds removed, thinly sliced lengthways

2 tbsp freshly snipped chives

Olive oil spray

250g steamed green beans

METHOD
STEP 1

Cut each breast into 3 thin escalopes, then toss in the combined paprika and cayenne to lightly coat. Set aside. Place avocado, lime, chili and chives in a bowl. Season and stir gently to combine. Set aside.

STEP 2

Heat a large frypan over high heat and spray with oil. Cook chicken, in 2 batches, for 2 minutes each side until cooked. Stand for 3 minutes, then halve each piece on an angle. Serve chicken on beans and salsa, and drizzle with any resting juices.

NUTRITION VALUE

1417 KJ Energy, 16g fat, 4g saturated fat, 4g fiber, 43g protein, 3g carbs.

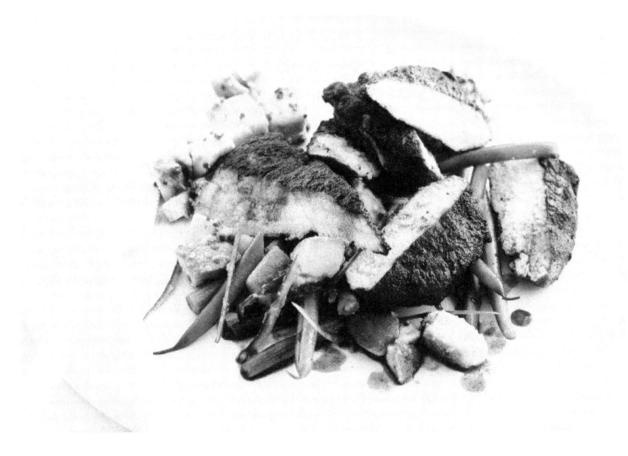

CHARGRILLED SWORDFISH WITH CAPER SALSA

Fish is packed with protein, plus it's a healthy choice for the family.

MAKES 4 SERVING/ TOTAL TIME 25 MINUTE

INGREDIENTS

4 (150g each) swordfish steaks

2 tsp olive oil

Crusty bread, to serve

CAPER SALSA

2 tbsp drained baby capers, roughly chopped

1 tbsp finely chopped fresh flat-leaf parsley leaves

1/2 tbsp lemon juice

1 1/2 tbsp olive oil

METHOD

STEP 1

Make caper salsa Combine capers, parsley, lemon juice and oil in a bowl.

STEP 2

Heat barbecue chargrill on medium heat. Brush both sides of fish with oil. Cook for 4 to 5 minutes each side or until just cooked through. Transfer to a glass or ceramic dish. Top with salsa. Cover. Set aside for 5 minutes to rest. Serve with bread.

NUTRITION VALUE

1559 KJ Energy, 20g fat, 5g saturated fat, 11.3g protein, 12g carbs.

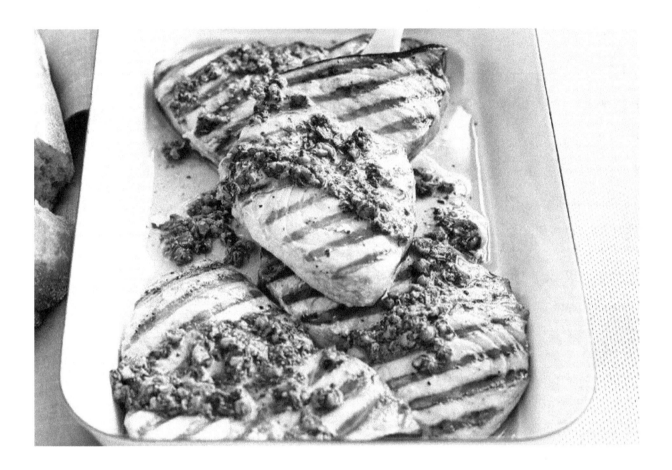

BARBECUED SALMON WITH LEMON AND HERBS

Whether you're having a weekend barbie, or planning a more casual Christmas, this **salmon** recipe could not be simpler.

MAKES 12 SERVING/ TOTAL TIME 4 HOUR 15 MINUTE

INGREDIENTS

1/2 cup olive oil

2 garlic cloves, finely chopped

2 lemons, juiced

2 tablespoons small capers, drained, chopped

1/3 cup dill leaves, finely chopped

1 bunch lemon thyme, roughly chopped

sea salt

12 x 180g Atlantic **salmon** fillets, skin on

lemon wedges, to serve

METHOD

STEP 1

Combine oil, garlic, 1/3 cup lemon juice, capers, dill and lemon thyme in a large jug. Season with sea salt and pepper. Place salmon, in a single layer, in a large ceramic dish. Pour over half the marinade. Turn salmon over and pour over remaining marinade. Cover. Refrigerate for 2 to 4 hours to marinate. Remove from fridge 30 minutes before cooking.

STEP 2

Preheat a greased barbecue plate on medium-high heat. Barbecue salmon, skin side up, for 3 minutes. Turn and barbecue, brushing occasionally with marinade, for 4 to 6 minutes (depending on thickness) or until just cooked through. Serve with lemon wedges.

NUTRITION VALUE

1484 KJ Energy, 19g fat, 5g saturated fat, 1g fiber, 44g protein, 1g carbs.

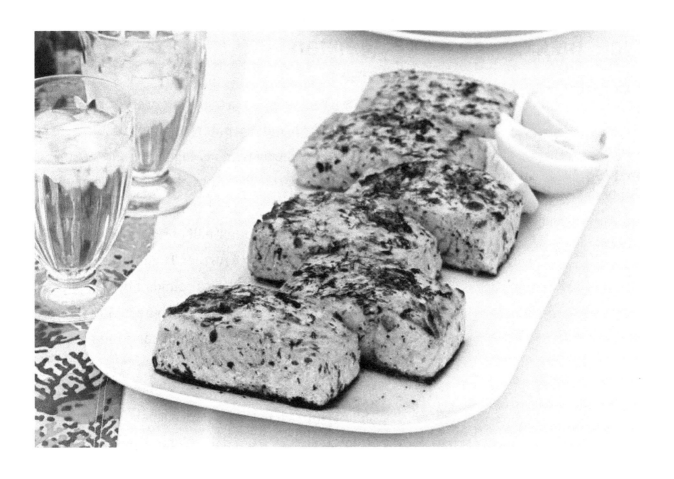

SALMON WITH SWEET POTATOES AND ZUCCHINI

Salmon is the star attraction of this very tasty dinner recipe.

MAKES 4 SERVING/ TOTAL TIME 55 MINUTE

INGREDIENTS

400g orange sweet potatoes (kumara)

Olive oil cooking spray

2 zucchinis

4 x 175g pieces **salmon**, pin-boned, skinned

80g pitted Sicilian green olives

1/2 bunch mint

60ml (1/4 cup) extra virgin olive oil

1 lemon

1 clove garlic

1/2 avocado

METHOD

STEP 1

Place a roasting pan in oven and preheat to 220C fan-forced. Wash and dry potatoes, then cut into 1cm cubes. Line hot oven tray with baking paper and scatter potatoes over one half. Spray with oil, season with salt and pepper, and roast for 10 minutes. Cut zucchinis into 1cm cubes. Add to other half of tray. Spray with oil, season and roast for a further 10 minutes, Spray salmon with oil and season. Place a round of baking paper in the base of a frying pan over high heat. Add salmon, curved-side down first, and cook for 3 minutes .

STEP 2

Meanwhile, to make salsa, place olives, mint and 2 tablespoons oil in the bowl of a small food processor. Squeeze in juice from half of lemon, peel and crush in garlic, then process until finely chopped Finely chop avocado and add to bowl, then season. Spoon remaining olive mixture over vegetables in pan, toss to combine, then divide among plates.

NUTRITION VALUE

2684 KJ Energy, 20g fat,
5g fiber, 46g protein, 15g carbs.

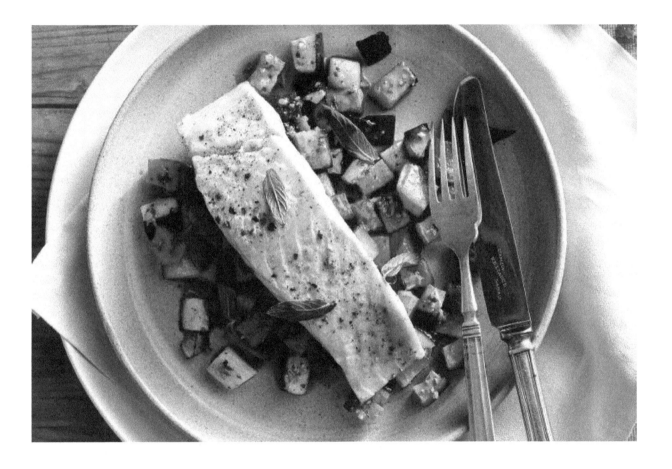

CHICKEN AND CAULIFLOWER FRIED 'RICE'

Cut back on your carbs without even noticing. This clever cauliflower fried rice is a winner for mid-week dinners.

MAKES 4 SERVING/ TOTAL TIME 40 MINUTE

INGREDIENTS

700g **cauliflower**, broken into florets

1 1/2 tablespoons peanut oil

2 eggs, lightly beaten

500g Lilydale Free Range Chicken Thigh, trimmed, cut into bite size pieces

1 cup corn kernels

2 garlic cloves, crushed

1 tablespoon finely grated ginger

3 green onions, thinly sliced

1 cup frozen peas, thawed

150g snow peas, trimmed, sliced on the diagonal

1 1/2 tablespoons tamari

1 long fresh red chili, thinly sliced

1/4 cup coarsely chopped coriander, plus extra sprigs to serve

METHOD

STEP 1

Heat 1/2 teaspoon of oil in a large wok over high heat. Pour half of egg, swirling wok to make a large omelets. Cook for 1 minute or until set. Flip onto a clean board, roll up tightly and thinly slice. Repeat with another ½ teaspoon of oil and remaining egg to make another omelets.

STEP 2

Heat 1 teaspoon of oil in same wok over medium-high heat. Stir-fry third of chicken for 3-4 minutes or until browned and cooked through. Repeat with another 2 teaspoons of oil and remaining chicken. Set aside. Heat remaining oil and stir-fry corn for 1 minute or until lightly charred. Add garlic, ginger and 2/3 of onion and stir-fry for 1-2 minutes or until fragrant and onion has softened. Add cauliflower, peas and snow peas and stir-fry for 3 minutes or until well coated and hot. Return chicken to the wok with sauce if using and stir-fry until hot. Serve topped with omelets, chili.

NUTRITION VALUE

1522 KJ Energy, 14.6g fat, 3.3g saturated fat, 8.7g fiber, 35.7g protein, 14.5g carbs.

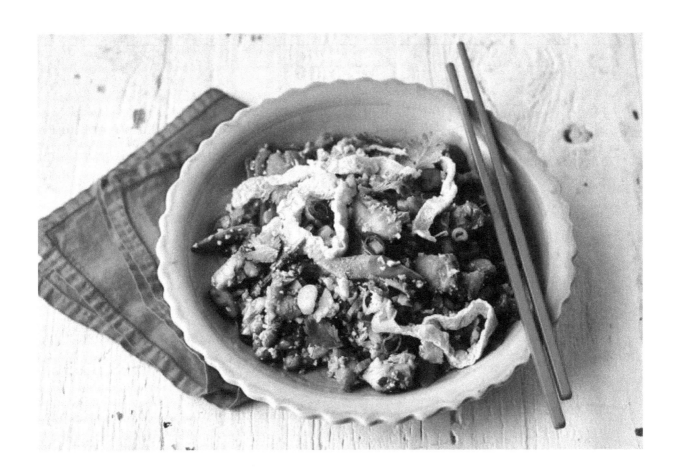

CURTIS STONE'S CAULIFLOWER FRIED RICE

We've swapped rice for cauliflower rice in this healthier cauliflower fried rice that's loaded with vegies.

MAKES 4 SERVING/ TOTAL TIME 20 MINUTE

INGREDIENTS

1/2 medium **cauliflower**, cored, coarsely chopped (about 480g)

2 extra-large Coles Australian Free-Range Eggs

2 tbs canola oil, divided

1 tbs sesame oil

100g snow peas, trimmed, thinly sliced lengthways

1 carrot, peeled, thinly sliced

5 spring onions, thinly sliced, white and pale green parts separated from dark green parts

1 tbs finely grated ginger

2 garlic cloves, crushed

2 tbs salt-reduced soy sauce

1/2 cup (75g) unsalted roasted cashews, coarsely chopped

METHOD

STEP 1

Pulse half the cauliflower in a food processor until very finely chopped. Don't overdo it or it will get mushy. Transfer to a bowl. Repeat with the remaining cauliflower .

STEP 2

Using a fork, whisk eggs in a bowl. Heat a large non-stick frying pan or wok over high heat. Add 1 tbs canola oil and egg. Cook for 30 secs or until almost set. Continue cooking, turning the egg and breaking into pieces, until cooked through. Transfer to a plate. Chop.

STEP 3

Add sesame oil and remaining canola oil to the pan or wok. Add the snow peas, carrot, white and pale green parts of the spring onions, ginger and garlic. Stir-fry for 1½ mins. Stir in the cauliflower rice and soy sauce. Cook, stirring often, for 2 mins ,Remove the pan or wok from heat and fold in the egg, dark green parts of the spring onions and cashews.

NUTRITION VALUE

1405 KJ Energy, 20g fat, 4g saturated fat, 7g fiber, 20g protein, 11g carbs.

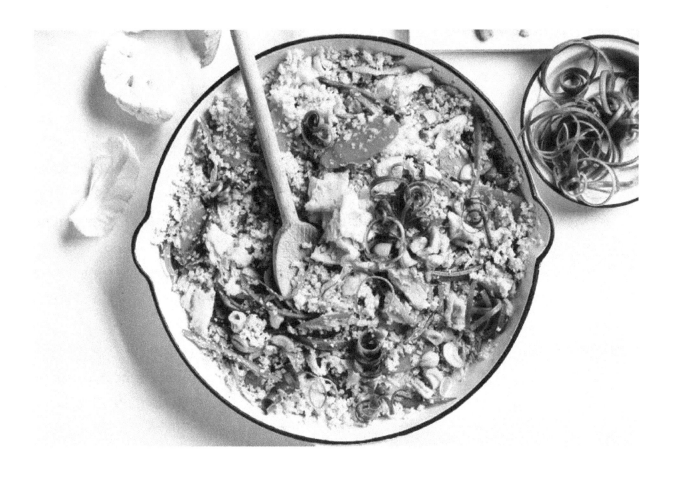

LITTLE PIES WITH SWEET POTATO TOPPING

Whip up an easy, healthy and delicious weeknight dinner with these simple little sweet **potato** pies.

MAKES 4 SERVING/ TOTAL TIME 65 MINUTE

INGREDIENTS

500g orange sweet potato, peeled, diced

2 teaspoons olive oil

1 small brown onion, finely chopped

1 small carrot, peeled, finely chopped

1 small zucchini, finely chopped

400g lean **beef mince**

400g can diced tomatoes

Mixed salad leaves, to serve

METHOD

STEP 1

Preheat oven to 200°C/ 180°C fan-forced. Cook potato in a large saucepan of boiling water for 15 minutes or until tender. Drain. Transfer to a bowl. Season with salt and pepper. Mash until smooth. Cover to keep warm.

STEP 2

Meanwhile, heat oil in a large saucepan over medium heat. Add onion, carrot and zucchini. Cook, stirring occasionally, for 5 to 6 minutes or until softened. Add mince. Cook, stirring with a wooden spoon to break up mince, for 3 to 4 minutes or until browned.

STEP 3

Add tomato. Stir to combine. Reduce heat to medium-low. Simmer for 5 to 10 minutes or until thickened. Spoon mixture into four 1 cup-capacity ovenproof dishes. Top each with potato.

STEP 4

Place dishes on a baking tray. Bake for 15 minutes or until golden and heated through. Serve with salad leaves.

NUTRITION VALUE

1175 KJ Energy, 9.5g fat, 3g saturated fat, 5g fiber, 25g protein, 13g carbs.

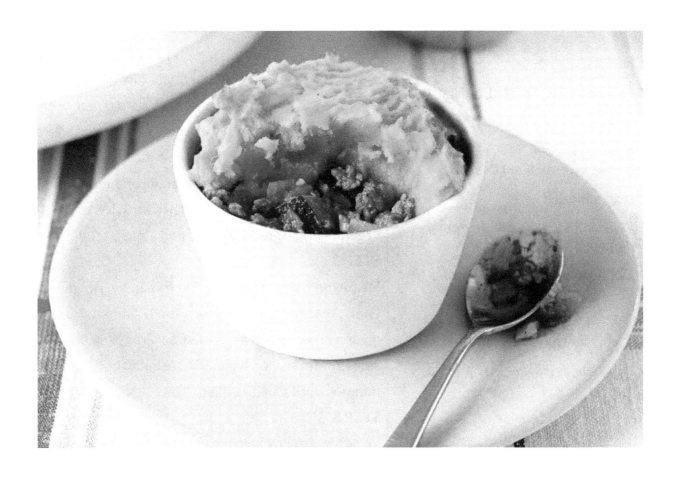

SUNDAY ROAST FISH

Feel like a Sunday roast without the meat? Do it with fish and your favorite vegies.

MAKES 4 SERVING/ TOTAL TIME 60 MINUTE

INGREDIENTS

1 bunch baby (Dutch) carrots, peeled

4 small parsnips, peeled, halved

8 garlic cloves (unpeeled)

4 rosemary sprigs, plus extra chopped rosemary (or parsley) to serve

2 tbsp olive oil

100g small shiitake **mushrooms**, trimmed

4 x 200g blue eye fillets (or other firm white fish)

16 baby brussels sprouts (or 8 small), halved, blanched for 2 minutes

2 tbsp balsamic vinegar (optional)

METHOD

STEP 1

Preheat the oven to 200C. Arrange carrots, parsnips, garlic and 4 rosemary sprigs in a roasting pan, then drizzle with 1 tablespoon oil and season. Toss well to combine, then bake for 20-25 minutes. Add mushrooms to pan, drizzle with 1 tablespoon oil and toss again. Bake for 15 minutes, turning once or twice, or until vegetables are golden brown and almost tender.

STEP 2

Meanwhile, heat a lightly oiled frypan over high heat. Cook the fish, skin-side down, for 1-2 minutes until golden and crisp. Transfer fish to a roasting pan, skin-side up, and season well. Add sprouts, then bake for 6-8 minutes until fish is cooked.

STEP 3

To serve, discard baked rosemary, then divide fish, vegetables and garlic among warm plates. Drizzle with balsamic if desired, then scatter with chopped rosemary or parsley. The garlic should be soft, ready to be squeezed out to mingle with the juices on the plate.

NUTRITION VALUE

1376 KJ Energy, 11g fat, 2g saturated fat, 7g fiber, 46g protein, 8g carbs.

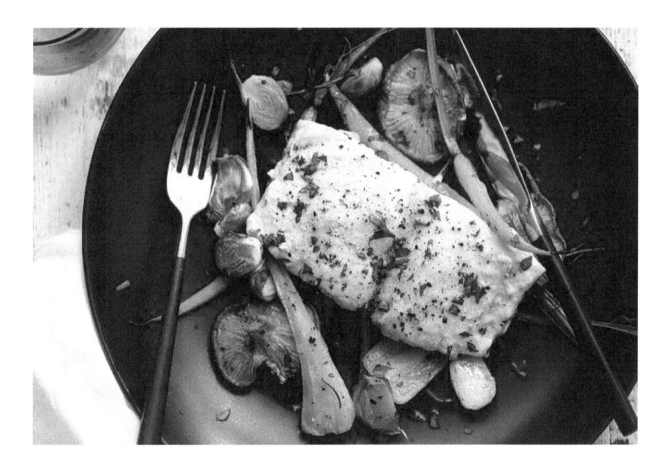

SALMON AND AVOCADO CEVICHE

This beautiful ceviche makes a colorful and elegant appetizer to your gourmet dinner feast.

MAKES 4 SERVING/ TOTAL TIME 55 MINUTE

INGREDIENTS

2 (about 400g) **salmon** fillets, skin removed, cut into 5mm pieces

1/3 cup (80ml) fresh lime juice

1 green Birdseye chili, seeded, finely chopped

1 red Birdseye chili, seeded, finely chopped

1 Spanish onion, finely chopped

1 just ripe avocado, halved, stoned, peeled, finely chopped

1 kaffir lime leaf, vein removed, finely shredded

1/4 cup freshly shredded coconut

Salmon roe, to serve

Baby salad leaves, to serve

METHOD

STEP 1

Combine the salmon, lime juice and combined chilies in a glass or ceramic bowl. Cover with plastic wrap and place in the fridge for 30 minutes to marinate.

STEP 2

Add the onion, avocado, kaffir lime and coconut. Gently toss mixture until just combined.

STEP 3

Place an 8cm pastry cutter on a serving plate. Spoon one quarter of the mixture into the pastry cutter and gently press with the back of a spoon. Remove the cutter. Repeat with remaining salmon mixture on serving dishes. Top with a small dollop of salmon roe and sprinkle with baby salad leaves, if desired.

NUTRITION VALUE

1505 KJ Energy, 20g fat, 5g saturated fat, 4g fiber, 26g protein, 2g carbs.

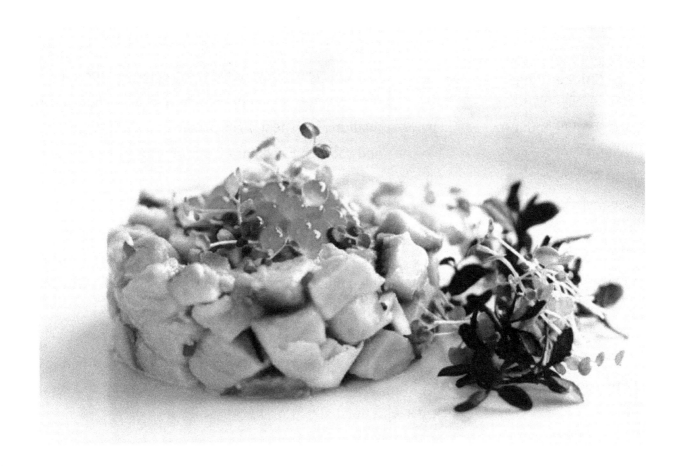

CHICKEN SOUP

Traditional chicken soup is said to cure the common cold. This healthy recipe uses lots of different herbs and spices to enhance the flavor.

MAKES 4 SERVING/ TOTAL TIME 55 MINUTE

INGREDIENTS

4 (about 900g) Lilydale Free Range **Chicken Thigh**, skinned, excess fat trimmed

1 large brown onion, halved, finely chopped

1 large carrot, peeled, finely chopped

1 celery stick, trimmed, finely chopped

2 large garlic cloves, finely chopped

2 tablespoons finely chopped fresh continental parsley stems

6 sprigs fresh thyme, leaves picked

2L (8 cups) water

1/2 teaspoon whole black peppercorns

Sea salt flakes

1/4 cup finely chopped fresh continental parsley, extra

METHOD

STEP 1

Combine chicken, onion, carrot, celery, garlic, parsley, thyme, water and peppercorns in a large saucepan over medium-high heat. Bring to the boil. Reduce heat to low and cook, covered, for 40 minutes or until vegetables are very tender.

STEP 2

Use tongs to transfer the chicken to a clean work surface. Hold with tongs and cut the chicken meat from the bones. Discard bones. Tear the chicken meat and add to the soup.

STEP 3

Taste and season with sea salt. Ladle soup among serving bowls. Sprinkle with extra parsley and serve immediately.

NUTRITION VALUE

1914 KJ Energy, 16.8g fat, 4.6g saturated fat, 1.9g fiber, 66.1g protein, 6.9g carbs.

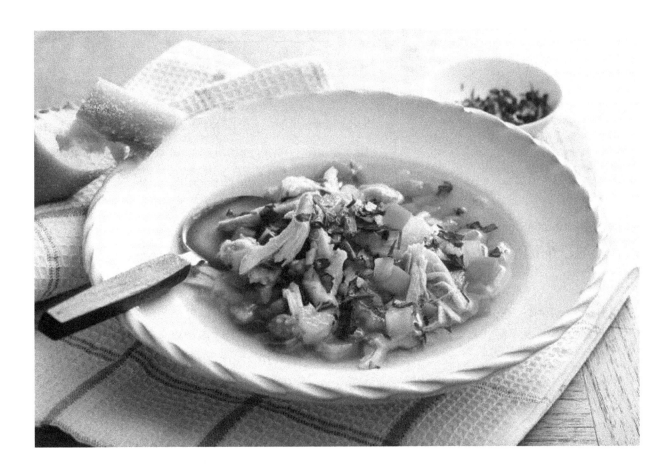

MACADAMIA-CRUSTED FISH WITH LEMON SPINACH

A crunchy coating of macadamia nuts turns fish fillets into a gourmet weeknight meal.

MAKES 4 SERVING/ TOTAL TIME 17 MINUTE

INGREDIENTS

1 lemon

190g (1 1/4 cups) macadamia nuts

1 tablespoon olive oil

1 tablespoon chopped fresh dill

1 garlic clove, crushed

4 firm white **fish fillets**

20g butter

300g baby spinach leaves

METHOD

STEP 1

Preheat oven to 180°C. Line a baking tray with non-stick baking paper. Finely grate the rind of the lemon. Cut the lemon in half and remove the seeds. Juice the lemon.

STEP 2

Place macadamia nuts in a mortar and crush with a pestle until they resemble coarse breadcrumbs. Stir in lemon rind, oil, dill and garlic. Season with salt and pepper. Place fish on the prepared tray. Divide macadamia nut mixture among the fish and press down firmly. Bake for 8-10 minutes or until fish flakes easily when tested with a fork in the thickest part.

STEP 3

Meanwhile, heat the butter in a frying pan over medium-high heat. Add the spinach and lemon juice. Cook, stirring, for 1-2 minutes or until the spinach wilts.

STEP 4

Divide the spinach among serving plates and top with the fish.

NUTRITION VALUE

1945 KJ Energy, 20g fat, 4g saturated fat, 5g fiber, 33g protein, 3g carbs.

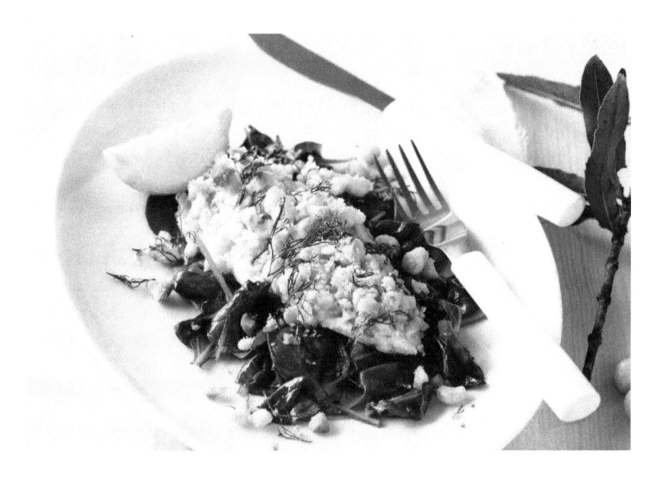

BEEF AND CASHEW STIR-FRY

This beef stir-fry is an easy-as family favorite dinner. With pre-marinated beef strips, cashews and broccoli, this flavor combo beats takeaway, any day. Serve with noodles, rice or naked as a paleo option.

MAKES 4 SERVING/ TOTAL TIME 20 MINUTE

INGREDIENTS

500g Coles Graze Grass Fed **Beef Stir-Fry strips**

1 red onion, cut into wedges

2 bunches baby broccoli, cut into 5cm lengths

1/3 cup (80ml) sweet chili sauce

1/2 cup (75g) toasted cashews

METHOD

STEP 1

Heat a non-stick wok over high heat. Add one-quarter of the beef and stir-fry for 1-2 mins or until browned. Transfer to a bowl.

STEP 2

Repeat in 3 more batches with remaining beef.

STEP 3

Add onion and baby broccoli to the wok and stir-fry for 2 mins or until just tender. Return the beef to the wok with sweet chili sauce and cashews. Stir-fry for 2 mins or until heated through.

NUTRITION VALUE

1586 KJ Energy, 16g fat, 4g saturated fat, 5g fiber, 32g protein, 14.6g carbs.

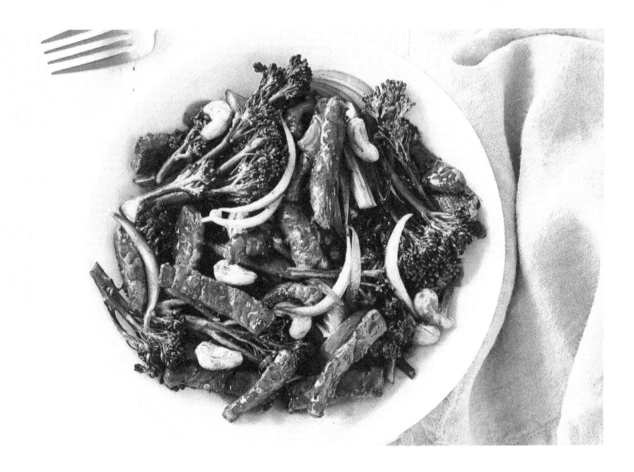

Desserts

CHOCOLATE SOUFFLE

This deep chocolate souffle is the perfect dessert for a romantic evening, or if you're just a chocolate lover looking for a quick fix. It's not loaded with refined sugar, but you wouldn't know it to taste it.

MAKES 2 SERVING/ TOTAL TIME 30 MINUTE

INGREDIENTS

2 tablespoons coconut oil plus more for greasing

1 tablespoon unsweetened cocoa powder

3 ounces chopped dark chocolate

1 teaspoon vanilla extract

1 tablespoon coconut milk

1 tablespoon honey

2 eggs separated

1/4 teaspoon sea salt

1/4 teaspoon cream of tartar

Serve with: coconut whipped cream or fresh berries

METHOD

STEP 1

Preheat oven to 375 degrees F.

Lightly grease 2 ramekins with coconut oil and dust with cocoa powder. Set on a baking sheet and set aside.

Put the chocolate and 2 tablespoons coconut oil in a microwave safe bowl and microwave in 15 second intervals until chocolate is melted, stirring each time. Let the chocolate mixture cool to the touch and whisk in the vanilla, coconut milk, honey, and egg yolks.

Put the egg whites in a mixing bowl with the salt and cream of tartar. Beat with a hand or stand mixer until you have stiff peaks.

STEP 2

Using a spatula, carefully fold the egg whites into the chocolate mixture. When they are just incorporated, divide the mixture between the ramekins.

Bake for 14-15 minutes until the souffles are set up in the middle. Take out of the oven and serve with whipped cream and berries if desired

NUTRITION VALUE

459 Kcal, 20g fat,
5g fiber, 21g protein, 13.9g carbs.

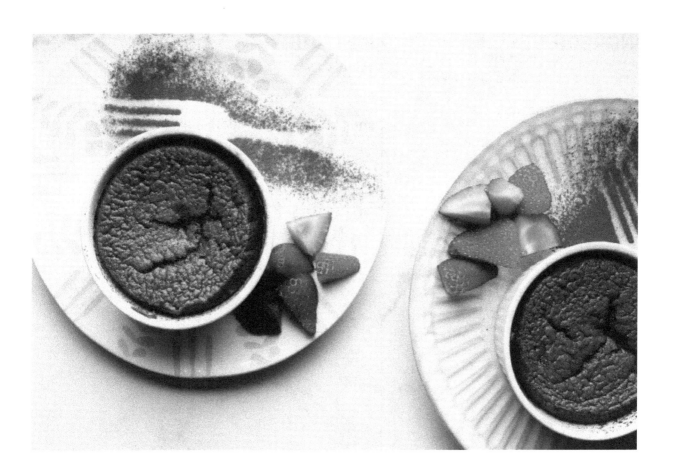

CHOCOLATE AVOCADO MOUSSE

You'll never know that the rich and creamy mousse you're eating is actually made of avocados. That means you get nutrients and good fats while also satisfying your sweet tooth.

MAKES 4 SERVING/ TOTAL TIME 30 MINUTE

INGREDIENTS

2 ripe avocados pitted and peeled

1/2 cup cocoa powder

3 tablespoons almond milk

1 teaspoon vanilla extract

1/4 teaspoon sea salt

1/4 cup honey

METHOD

STEP 1

Put all of the ingredients in a blender or food processor and process until smooth and creamy.

Serve immediately.

NUTRITION VALUE	213 Kcal, 12g fat, 9g fiber, 21g protein, 14g carbs.

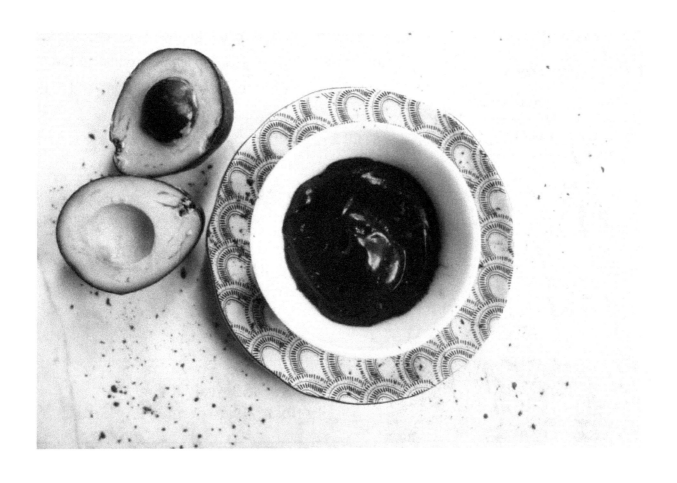

CHOCOLATE ICE CREAM

Creamy and decadent, this proves you don't have to give up ice cream to eat a healthy diet.

MAKES 4 SERVING/ TOTAL TIME 8 HOUR 30 MINUTE

INGREDIENTS

2 cans full-fat coconut milk, refrigerated overnight or 1 can coconut cream

1/4 cup honey

1/2 cup cocoa powder

2 tablespoons coconut oil

1 tablespoon vanilla extra

1/2 teaspoon sea salt

METHOD

STEP 1

Open the cans of coconut milk and remove the cream that has formed at the top, leaving the liquid. Add it to a blender.

In a small saucepan, combine the honey, cocoa, coconut oil, vanilla, and salt. Heat on low and whisk until smooth. Turn off heat, let cool slightly, and add to the blender with the cream.

STEP 2

Blend until smooth and creamy.

Transfer this mixture to an ice cream maker and follow the manufacturer's instructions to churn and transfer to freezer.

Freeze for several hours before serving.

NUTRITION VALUE	459 Kcal, 20g fat, 4g fiber, 20g protein, 14.2g carbs.

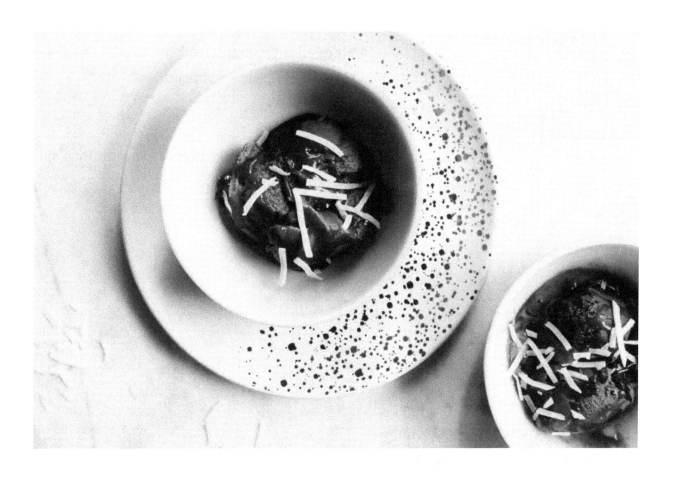

CHOCOLATE COCONUT FUDGE

If you're a chocoholic, this easy fudge recipe is perfect for you. Store it in the freezer for an anytime treat.

MAKES 16 SERVING/ TOTAL TIME 20 MINUTE

INGREDIENTS

1/2 cup coconut oil

1/2 cup creamy almond butter

1/2 cup cocoa powder

1/4 cup honey

Coarse sea salt

METHOD

STEP 1

Line a square baking dish with parchment paper. Combine all of the ingredients in a small saucepan over low heat and whisk until smooth.

STEP 2

Pour the mixture into the prepared baking dish and refrigerate for at least 2 hours.

Cut into squares and serve. Store leftovers in the fridge or freezer.

NUTRITION VALUE	130 Kcal, 11g fat, 2g fiber, 20g protein, 8g carbs.

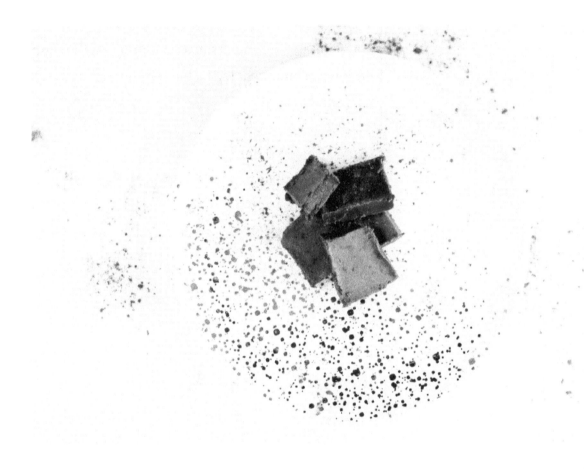

CARROT CAKE BITES

With no cooking required, these bite sized treats give you something sweet after a meal without the heaviness that comes from traditional carrot cake.

MAKES 24 SERVING/ TOTAL TIME 20 MINUTE

INGREDIENTS

2 carrots diced

1 cup chopped dates

2 cups walnuts

1 cup unsweetened coconut flakes

1 teaspoon cinnamon

2 tablespoons maple syrup

1 teaspoon vanilla extract

1 tablespoon almond butter

1/2 teaspoon sea salt

METHOD

STEP 1

Put all of the ingredients in a food processor and pulse until well combined. Line a baking sheet with parchment paper.

STEP 2

Using a cookie scoop, scoop rounded balls onto the sheet pan. Roll into tight balls, and refrigerate for about an hour before serving.

Store remaining balls in an airtight container in the fridge.

NUTRITION VALUE

98 Kcal, 10g fat,
2g fiber, 20g protein, 7g carbs.

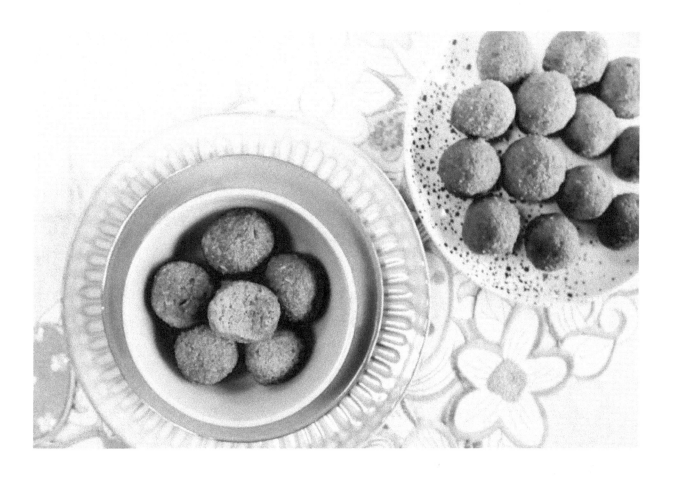

BAKED APPLES

So, few ingredients make a super healthy dessert. Perfect for chilly nights when you want a taste of fall without having to feel bad about it.

MAKES 2 SERVING/ TOTAL TIME 40 MINUTE

INGREDIENTS

2 apples

2 tablespoons maple syrup

1 teaspoon cinnamon

1/4 cup finely chopped walnuts

1/4 teaspoon sea salt

METHOD

STEP 1

Preheat oven to 375 degrees F.

Cut the apples in half and scoop out the core and seeds using a spoon or melon baller. Lay in baking dish cut side up.

STEP 2

Mix the maple syrup, cinnamon, walnuts, and salt in a small bowl until combined. Spread this mixture evenly over the apple halves.

Bake for 20-30 minutes until apples are tender and fragrant.

Serve warm.

NUTRITION VALUE

233 Kcal, 10g fat,
7g fiber, 20g protein, 14g carbs.

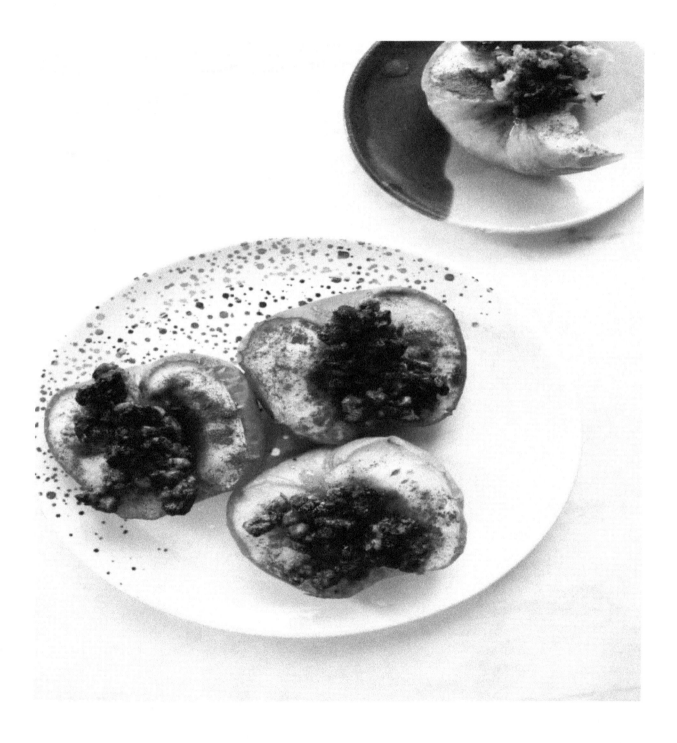

Snacks

"BREADED" PALEO CHICKEN CUTLETS {WHOLE30}

Crispy "breaded" Paleo Chicken Cutlets that are super easy and just as good as the original. Whole30 compliant, kid friendly!

MAKES 6 SERVING/ TOTAL TIME 15 MINUTE

INGREDIENTS

1.5 lbs. boneless skinless chicken breasts, thin sliced or pounded to 1/2" thickness
1 cup blanched almond flour*
1/4 cup coconut flour*
1 and 1/4 tsp fine grain sea salt
1/8 tsp black pepper
2 tsp Italian seasoning blend <--My favorite
1 tsp onion powder
1/2 tsp garlic powder
dash red pepper flakes optional
1 egg whisked
3 tbsp coconut oil + 2 tbsp ghee for frying**

METHOD
STEP 1
Mix all the dry ingredients in a medium shallow bowl (you will dredge the cutlets in the mixture)
Have your whisked egg in a shallow bowl, heat a large, heavy, deep skillet over medium heat and add 3 tbsp total of cooking fat (a combination of ghee and coconut oil, or all coconut.) Depending on the size of your skillet, you might have to fry these in 2 batches, so have additional cooking fat ready in case you need more.
STEP 2
Once the skillet it preheated (you can see if a drop of the dry mixture sizzles), dip one cutlet in the egg, shaking off excess, then coat in the dry mixture, shaking off excess. Place the chicken in the pan, then repeat the process for each piece of chicken.
Cook on one side until medium-golden brown (2 minutes) and crisp, then carefully turn over the chicken with tongs and cook the second side until golden brown and juices run clear, about 2 minutes depending on the thickness of your chicken***
Carefully remove chicken cutlets from skillet with tongs and place on a paper-towel lined plate to absorb excess grease. Serve hot with baked fries, sweet potatoes, or butternut squash fries! Enjoy!

NUTRITION VALUE

334 cal, 20g fat, 5g saturated fat, 3g fiber, 29g protein, 7g carbs.

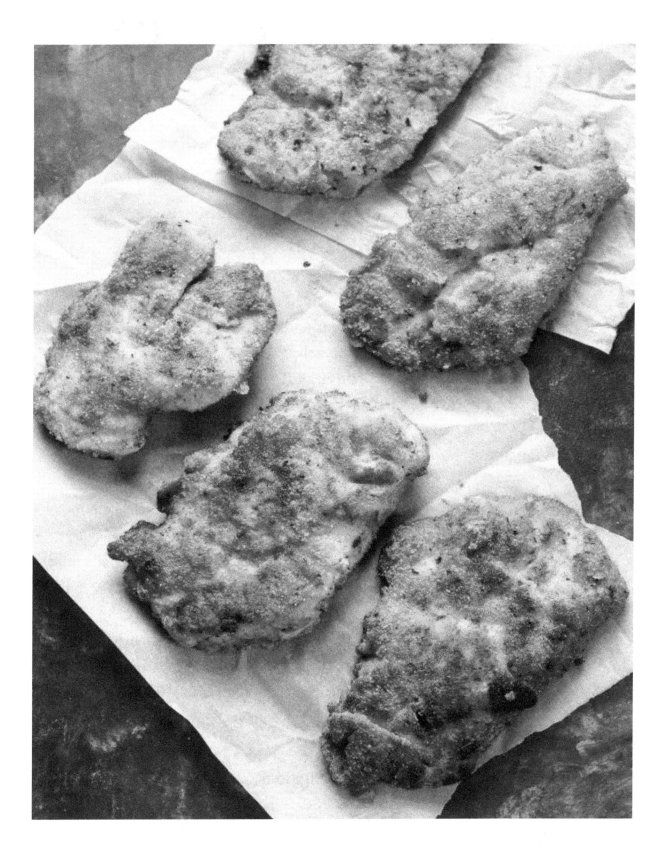

CREAMY POTATO CHOWDER WITH SHRIMP AND BACON

This one-pot Creamy Potato Chowder with Shrimp and Bacon is the ultimate comfort food on a chilly evening!

MAKES 6 SERVING/ TOTAL TIME 40 MINUTE

INGREDIENTS

1 package nitrate-free bacon
1-pound deveined shrimp
1 onion, minced
2 garlic cloves
3 Yukon potatoes, diced
2 celery ribs, diced
2 carrots, minced
1/4 teaspoon sweet paprika
1/2 teaspoon dried thyme
4 cups chicken stock
1 cup fresh or frozen corn, thawed and cooked
1/4 cup heavy cream or ¼ cup cashew cream
1 tablespoon fresh parsley, for garnish
1 sprig fresh thyme, for garnish
1 tablespoon scallions, for garnish

METHOD

STEP 1

Heat a large Dutch oven over medium heat. Add bacon and cook until crispy, around 5-8 minutes. Turn off heat and place bacon on a plate lined with paper towels. Drain all but 1 tablespoon of bacon fat out of the pan. Turn heat to medium-high and cook shrimp for about 2-3 minutes on each side, or until pink and fully cooked through.

STEP 2

Place garlic and onion into the Dutch oven. Cook for 1-2 minutes or until onions start to turn translucent. Add potato, celery, and carrots to the pot. Cook until potato starts to soften. Add in spices. Cook for 1-2 minutes, making sure to scrape up all of the brown bits from the bottom of the pan. Cover and bring to a boil over medium-high heat. Once at a boil, add corn and turn down heat and let simmer for 10-15 minutes. Serve in desired serving bowls.

NUTRITION VALUE

266 cal, 11.4g fat, 3.8g saturated fat, 3g fiber, 23.7g protein, 14g carbs.

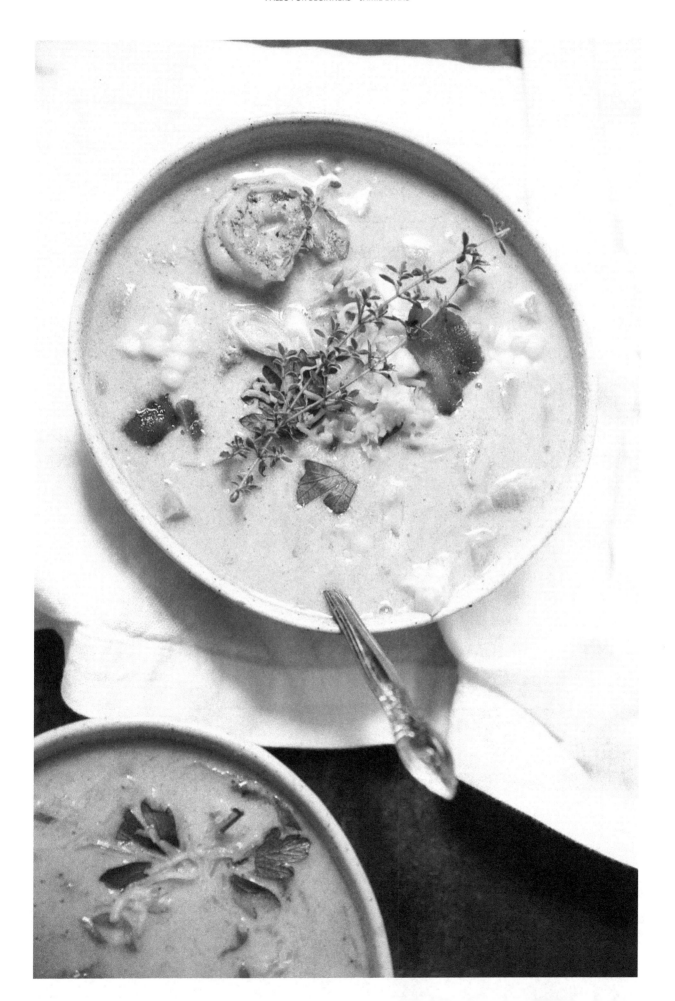

CREAM OF ZUCCHINI SOUP

An easy summer soup that will use up a bountiful of zucchini if you have them. It can be served chilled or hot, so be sure to try both ways!

MAKES 4 SERVING/ TOTAL TIME 20 MINUTE

INGREDIENTS

1 tablespoon olive oil

1 onion diced

4 zucchini diced

2 cloves garlic minced

1 teaspoon dried thyme

1 cup chicken broth

1 cup heavy cream

Fresh chopped basil leaves for serving

Sea salt and fresh ground pepper to taste

METHOD

STEP 1

Heat the oil in a pot and add the onions, zucchini, garlic, and thyme. Cook until softened and add the broth. Bring to a boil, and simmer for 5 minutes.

STEP 2

Transfer to a blender and blend until smooth; add back to the pot and add the cream. Simmer for 5 minutes. Serve topped with the basil.

NUTRITION VALUE

289 Kcal, 20g fat,
3g fiber, 20g protein, 11g carbs.

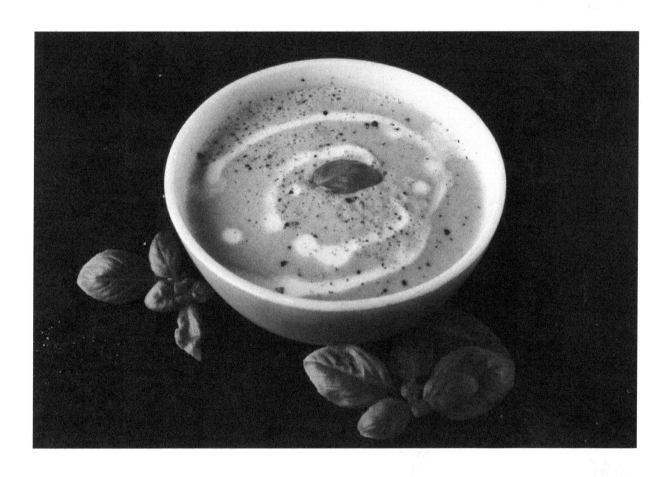

SHRIMP AND VEGGIE CHOWDER

An easy and healthy soup that is creamy and delicious. Full of protein and fiber, it will become a regular on your dinner table.

MAKES 4 SERVING/ TOTAL TIME 20 MINUTE

INGREDIENTS

1 tablespoon olive oil

1 pound shrimp chopped

1 onion diced

2 stalks celery diced

1 bell pepper diced

2 cloves garlic minced

1 carrot diced

1 zucchini diced

1 tablespoon Old Bay seasoning

2 cups chicken broth

1 cup heavy cream or coconut milk

Sea salt and fresh ground pepper to taste

METHOD

STEP 1

Heat the oil in a large pot. Add the shrimp and cook until pink. Remove from pot.

STEP 2

Add the veggies and Old Bay and cook until softened and lightly browned. Add the broth and cream and bring to a low simmer.

Simmer for 10-15 minutes, and add the shrimp back to the pot. Heat through and serve.

NUTRITION VALUE

421 Kcal, 20g fat, 2g fiber, 32g protein, 9g carbs.

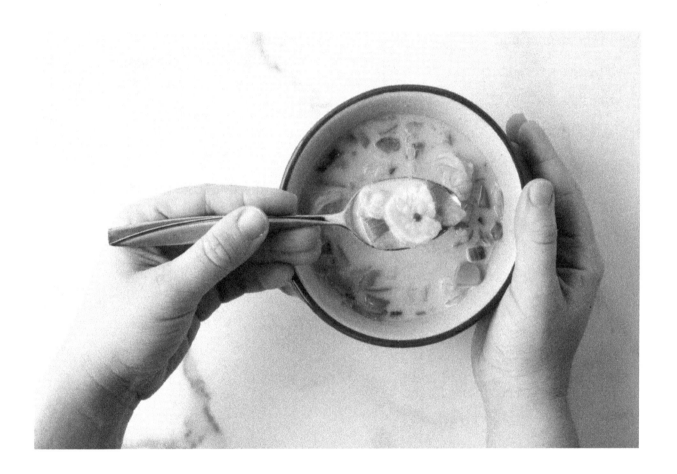

CHICKEN FAJITA SOUP

Made with chicken thighs for richer flavor, this easy to make soup will satisfy your cravings for fajitas but without all the carbs!

MAKES 4 SERVING/ TOTAL TIME 30 MINUTE

INGREDIENTS

1 tablespoon olive oil

3 bell peppers sliced

1 onion sliced

2 cloves garlic minced

1 teaspoon cumin

1 teaspoon chili powder

1 teaspoon oregano

1 teaspoon paprika

4 chicken thighs

6 cups chicken broth

Juice of 1 lime

Chopped cilantro diced avocado, sour cream, for serving

Sea salt and fresh ground pepper to taste

METHOD

STEP 1

Heat the oil in a large pot. Add the peppers, onions, garlic, and seasonings. Cook until softened and add the chicken and broth.

STEP 2

Bring to a boil and reduce to a simmer. Simmer until chicken is cooked through. Remove and let cool slightly. Shred and add back to the pot.

Add the lime juice and simmer for 5 minutes.

Serve topped with desired accompaniments.

NUTRITION VALUE

331 Kcal, 18g fat,
2g fiber, 26g protein, 8g carbs.

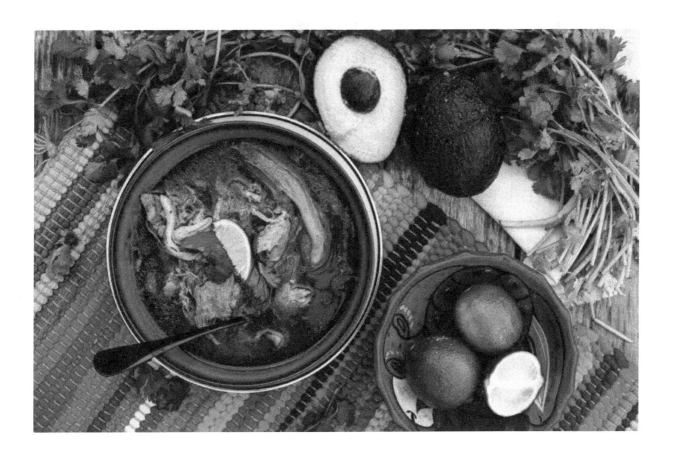

CAULIFLOWER SHAKSHUKA

Shakshuka is an easy dish to make when you want to impress, but it's also nutritious and delicious. This version, with the addition of cauliflower is hearty and filling. This is the perfect healthy brunch recipe for lazy weekends.

MAKES 2 SERVING/ TOTAL TIME 20 MINUTE

INGREDIENTS

2 tablespoons olive oil

1 onion chopped

1 cup cauliflower florets

3 cloves garlic minced

2 tablespoons tomato paste

1 teaspoon ground cumin

1/2 teaspoon smoked paprika

1 28- ounce can crushed tomatoes

6 large eggs

2 ounces crumbled feta

2 tablespoons chopped fresh parsley

Sea salt and fresh ground pepper to taste

METHOD

STEP 1

Preheat oven to 350 degrees F.

In a large straight sided skillet or braising pan, heat the oil. Add the onion and cauliflower and cook until soft and lightly browned. Add the garlic, tomato paste, and seasonings and cook for another minute. Add the tomatoes.

STEP 2

Make six small wells in the tomatoes and crack the eggs into each one. Season with salt and pepper and top with the feta.

Bake for 10-15 minutes, until egg whites are set and yolks are slightly firm. Remove from oven and sprinkle with parsley before serving.

NUTRITION VALUE

616 Kcal, 20g fat,
14g fiber, 32g protein, 14.9g carbs.

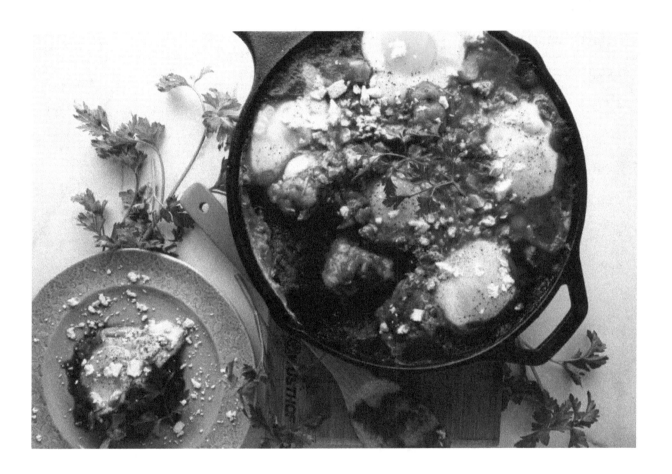

PUMPKIN SPICED PALEO GRANOLA

Eat with almond milk and fruit, or sprinkle a bit on top of high-quality yogurt. It also makes a delicious and addictive snack.

MAKES 12 SERVING/ TOTAL TIME 45 MINUTE

INGREDIENTS

1/8 cup coconut oil melted

1/4 cup honey

1/2 cup pecans

1/2 cup walnuts

1/2 cup sliced almonds

1/2 cup unsweetened coconut flakes

1/2 cup sunflower seeds

1/2 cup pumpkin seeds

3 tablespoons sesame seeds

3 tablespoons flax seeds

1 tablespoon pumpkin pie spice or season to taste

1/2 teaspoon sea salt

1/2 cup dried cranberries

METHOD

STEP 1

Preheat oven to 350 degrees F.

Combine the coconut oil and honey in a large bowl and whisk until combined. Add the nuts, seeds, pumpkin pie spice, and salt, and stir to coat well.

STEP 2

Spread mixture on a parchment or foil lined baking sheet. Bake for 30-40 minutes, until brown and fragrant. Remove from oven and stir in the cranberries. Let cool, then break up, or put in a food processor and pulse for a more traditional granola like texture.

This recipe makes about 4 cups. Store in an airtight container.

NUTRITION VALUE	245 Kcal, 18g fat, 3g fiber, 20g protein, 15g carbs.

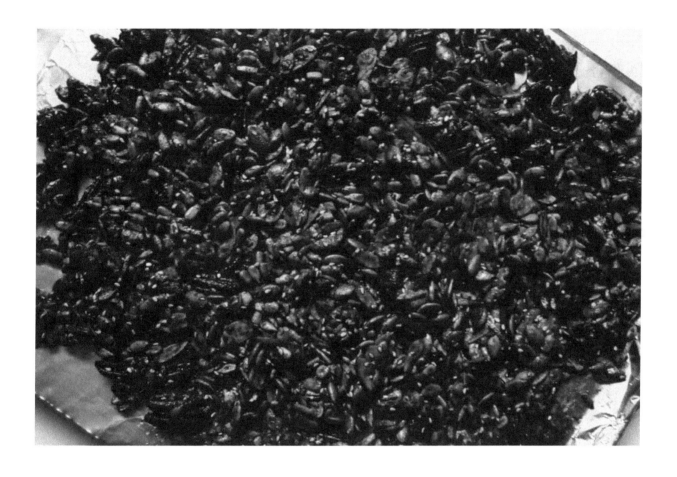

CHILI ROASTED CASHEWS

In addition to a simple snack, you can throw these chili roasted cashews in a salad, sprinkle on soup, or add to a stir-fry.

MAKES 8 SERVING/ TOTAL TIME 45 MINUTE

INGREDIENTS

2 cups raw cashews

1 tablespoon light olive oil

2 teaspoon chili powder

1 teaspoon honey

Juice of 1 lime

1/2 teaspoon sea salt

METHOD

STEP 1

Preheat oven to 350 degrees Line a baking sheet with parchment paper.

Put all of the ingredients in a freezer bag and shake until cashews are well coated. Spread evenly on the baking sheet.

STEP 2

Bake for 20-25 minutes until cashews are golden and fragrant. Allow to cool completely before serving. Store in an airtight container.

NUTRITION VALUE

181Kcal, 14g fat,
1g fiber, 19.9g protein, 10g carbs.

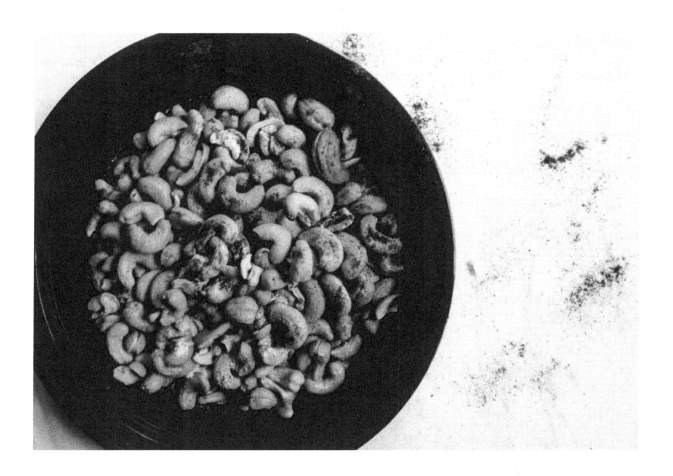

GUACAMOLE DEVILED EGGS

Deviled eggs get a redo with creamy avocado and fresh salsa. Make up a batch and then grab a couple when you need a quick snack.

MAKES 1 2 SERVING/ TOTAL TIME 20 MINUTE

INGREDIENTS

6 hardboiled eggs

1 avocado pitted and peeled

1 clove garlic minced

1/2 small tomato diced

1 tablespoon minced jalapeno

2 tablespoons red onion diced

2 tablespoons chopped cilantro

Juice of 1 lime

Sea salt and fresh ground pepper to taste

METHOD

STEP 1

Peel the hardboiled eggs and remove the yolks. Add them to a bowl with the avocado and mash.
Add the remaining ingredients and mix well.

STEP 2

Spoon the mixture into the egg white halves. If saving for later, put the guacamole mixture in an airtight container and spoon into the eggs when ready to eat.

NUTRITION VALUE	62 Kcal, 4g fat, 1g fiber, 4g protein, 2g carbs.

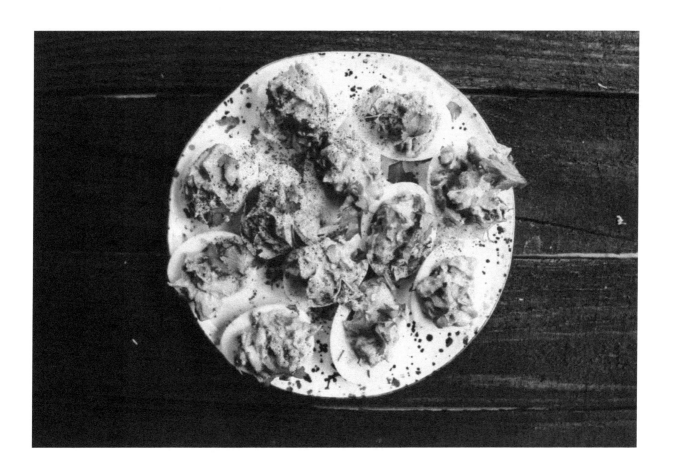

COCONUT CREAMED CUCUMBERS

The coconut milk and cucumbers in this easy side dish get a punch of heat from the pepper. This easy summer side dish is great for a backyard barbecue.

MAKES 4 SERVING/ TOTAL TIME 30 MINUTE

INGREDIENTS

2 cucumbers sliced

1/2 cup coconut milk

1 teaspoon lemon juice

1 teaspoon fresh ground black pepper

1 teaspoon fresh chopped dill

Sea salt to taste

METHOD

STEP 1
Combine all of the ingredients in a large bowl. Let stand at room temperature for 20 minutes or so to develop the flavors. Serve at room temperature or chilled.

NUTRITION VALUE

653 Kcal, 9g fat,
8g fiber, 46g protein, 14g carbs.

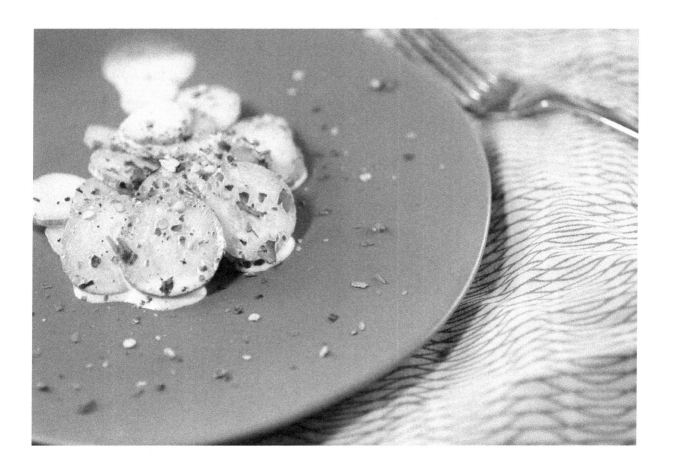

HOT PEPPER ROASTED BROCCOLI

Broccoli is one of those veggies that takes on new life when roasted in a hot oven. The edges become crisp, and the flavor comes alive in a way that it doesn't when steamed.

MAKES 4 SERVING/ TOTAL TIME 40 MINUTE

INGREDIENTS

1 head broccoli cut into florets

3 tablespoons olive oil

1 teaspoon crushed red pepper flakes

Juice of 1 lemon

Sea salt and fresh ground pepper to taste

METHOD

STEP 1

Preheat oven to 425 degrees F.

Toss all of the ingredients until broccoli is well coated, and spread evenly on a baking sheet.

Roast for 30-40 minutes, stirring once or twice, until broccoli is charred and tender. Serve immediately.

NUTRITION VALUE	467 Kcal, 20g fat, 1g fiber, 48.1g protein, 3.4g carbs.

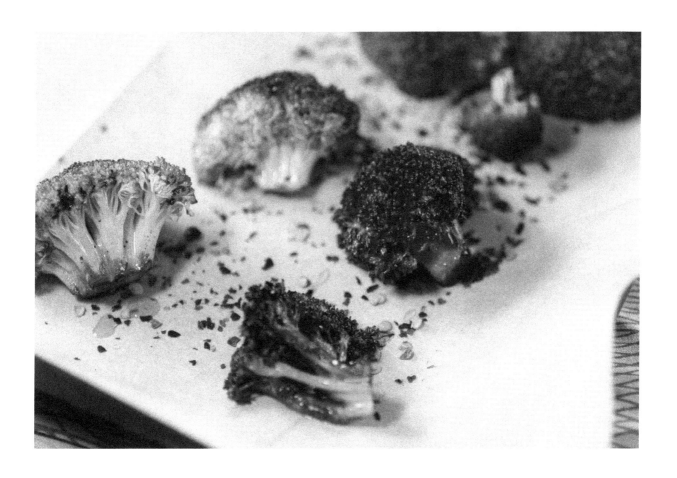

CPSIA information can be obtained
at www.ICGtesting.com
Printed in the USA
BVHW060158250621
610373BV00007B/1738